CYBERSECURITY FOR eHEALTH

CYBERSECURITY FOR eHEALTH

A Simplified Guide to Practical Cybersecurity for Non-Technical Healthcare Stakeholders & Practitioners

Emmanuel C. Ogu

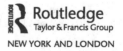
Routledge
Taylor & Francis Group

NEW YORK AND LONDON

First Edition published 2022
by Routledge
605 Third Avenue, New York, NY 10158

and by Routledge
2 Park Square, Milton Park, Abingdon, Oxon, OX14 4RN

Routledge is an imprint of the Taylor & Francis Group, an informa business

© 2022 Taylor & Francis Group, LLC

Library of Congress Cataloging-in-Publication Data
A catalog record for this title has been requested

ISBN: 978-1-032-18417-3 (hbk)
ISBN: 978-1-032-13904-3 (pbk)
ISBN: 978-1-003-25441-6 (ebk)

DOI: 10.1201/9781003254416

Typeset in Caslon
by SPi Technologies India Pvt Ltd (Straive)

To the **God** I serve – Giver of all wisdom and understanding.

To **Lyndar** and **Patra,** for bearing with the many weeks that I remained distracted from Family realities, while trying to focus on writing.

Contents

Preface

The modern realities of cybersecurity have uncovered the unpreparedness of many sectors and industries to deal with emerging trends. One of these sectors is the healthcare industry, a sector wherein the pervasiveness and proliferation of various eHealth innovations, systems, and applications in global healthcare, powered by modern information and communications technologies, have created a threat domain wherein policy and regulation struggle to keep pace with development, standardization faces several contextual challenges, and technical capacity is largely deficient. The spates of high-profile cyber incidents that have continued to unsettle the global healthcare sector suggest that this level of unpreparedness tends to have pervaded the entire apparatus, ranks, and file of healthcare organizations, even though the impact of such incidents, when measured by acceptable financial and reputational indices, have continued to remain calamitous.

As the rubber meets the road, it becomes necessary to synthesize the most-relevant and rudimentary knowledge pertaining to the realities of global cybersecurity as it relates to the healthcare sector and to present this knowledge in a form adapted to the technical incapacities of the stakeholders that work in the global healthcare industry. More so, a number of existing resources in this domain have been criticised for being either too technical in their content to be a useful and informative resource for non-technical healthcare stakeholders, or being too theoretical in its scope to present relevance for engaging with the practical realities of cybersecurity in the healthcare sector.

Thus, in this book, I have attempted to blend the integrity of the scientific approach to evidence-based discussions that define the academic character, with the quality of attention to detail and critical appraisal that distinguishes the native approach of the industry professional. It distills the most foundational information, and presents it in a compact manner that can be easily assimilated. This is achieved by drawing lessons from real-life case studies across the global healthcare industry to drive home otherwise complex principles and insights; especially for healthcare stakeholders without formal technical training in the workings of healthcare information and communication technologies. At the same time, it tries not to trivialize the critical discourse that is Cybersecurity, and the crucial implications that it portends for eHealth.

By excluding the hard-core technical stuff, I have managed to consolidate the more critical panels of focus, as a quick primer to enable non-technical healthcare stakeholders (*viz.*, medical professionals, healthcare workers, regulatory and compliance agencies, health centre managers, administrators & insurers, clients/patients, and third-party vendors) understand and deal more knowledgeably and effectively with the realities of cybersecurity for eHealth.

In summary, this book presents the basics of cybersecurity and an overview of eHealth, covering the foundational concepts, perspectives, and applications of cybersecurity in the context of eHealth. It goes on to present an in-depth traverse of the cybersecurity threat landscape to eHealth, discussing threat categories, threat agents, threat objectives, strategies and approaches featured by various threat agents, predisposing risk factors in cybersecurity threat situations, as well as the various tools/techniques that are deployed in cybersecurity incidents against eHealth. Further, it discusses approaches and best practices for enhancing personal cybersecurity as custodians of eHealth systems, services, and infrastructures – including an approach to progressively developing and sharpening an intuition for cybersecurity.

In addition, this book also presents the foundational principles of data and information security for eHealth deployments, covering the invariants of preserving integrity, safeguarding privacy, ensuring confidentiality, and guaranteeing availability. It then goes on to discuss physical, logical, and operational imperatives for securing eHealth systems and infrastructures, while also ensuring compliance through various monitoring and evaluation procedures and approaches in real-life ecosystems of eHealth deployments.

Finally, this book presents some thoughts on governance, ethics, and regulation in eHealth, highlighting notable international legislations that help to provide the necessary context for understanding the goals and challenges of regulation, as well as the roles and responsibilities of management/administration, and the relationship between compliance and security. It closes with an extensive glossary of definitions for key terms and words that feature within the book, as have been adjudged to be necessary to help boost a deeper understanding of the context and usage of these words for readers who do not have a technical background in Information Technology.

So, here! I present to you: *Cybersecurity for eHealth*.

– Emmanuel C. Ogu

Acknowledgement

I acknowledge the many healthcare stakeholders and professionals who have participated in my training and consultancy events over the past few years. Engaging and interacting with you provided much of the insight and context that helped inform the discussions within this book. I am grateful for the opportunity to learn from your various experiences across the global healthcare industry.

I also acknowledge my friend Yushavia and the remarkable team at Trishula Pathways and the African Healthcare Portal (AHP), whose push, partnership, and collaboration in the midst of a global lockdown occasioned by a rampaging pandemic, helped inspire the needed urgency that drove the development process of this book to completion within the shortest possible time.

Finally, I acknowledge the editorial leadership of John and the editorial support of Stephanie, both of whom helped make the publication process an all-around enjoyable experience.

Thank you!

– Emmanuel C. Ogu

Author Bio

Emmanuel C. Ogu is a Consummate Computer Scientist, a Chartered IT Professional, an Advocate for Digital Rights & Freedom, a Cybersecurity Specialist, a Technology Governance & Digital Development Expert, and a Sustainable Development Researcher. He is a 2020 Youth Ambassador of the Internet Society (ISOC) to the Internet Governance Forum (IGF), with more than 7 years of cumulative experience working at the intersection of Cybersecurity and Information Technology within the domains of Public Policy, Sustainable Development, and Internet Governance.

1
CYBERSECURITY BASICS & OVERVIEW OF eHEALTH

Introduction

In July of 2018, Singapore's Ministry of Health, and Cyber Security Agency received a report regarding a data breach at the Singapore General Hospital (SingHealth) – Singapore's largest group of healthcare institutions. This breach resulted in the stealing of 1.5 million records of personal data over a week-long period, and further targeted outpatient medication information of some 160,000 patients.

These patients were individuals who had visited specialist outpatient clinics and polyclinics at SingHealth from May 01, 2015, to Jul 04, 2018, and included the Prime Minister of Singapore – Lee Hsien Loong – as well as other senior ministers. It was to go down the memory lane as the *SingHealth* data breach. A high-profile cyber-attack that could have been prevented through better cybersecurity hygiene and practices, and occurred at a time when health data sold for at least $50 on the global black market. The *SingHealth* data breach uncovered a host of technical and non-technical lapses in the cybersecurity frameworks at SingHealth; and, an attacker that has been described as stealthy, "skilled, patient, and persistent" is believed to have orchestrated this breach[1].

At first, the Integrated Health Information System (IHIS) – the Agency responsible for the security of information technologies used in Singapore's public health system – detected the breach, following the recording of suspicious activity on one of the database servers that hosted electronic health records (EHRs). Initial investigations revealed that a malware infiltration on one of the front-end user workstations might have provided the entry point for the infamous attack, through which the masterminds were able to gain privileged access to server resources and equally mask their digital footprints properly.

DOI: 10.1201/9781003254416-1

In January 2019, an independent 450-page Report[2] of the high-level Committee of Inquiry (CoI) that was convened to investigate the incident, was published. Among several lapses and failures, this Report emphasized a lack of preparedness, proactiveness, and strategic foresight on the part of network security administrators. It also underscored insufficiencies in the regimen of the IHIS for cybersecurity awareness and training. Also highlighted was the naiveness on the part of system users who happened not to be familiar with basic cybersecurity practices, as well as security policies at SingHealth. The Report further spotlighted the existence of critical vulnerabilities in SingHealth's systems and infrastructure that made infiltration and unauthorized access relatively easier.

In summary, the Report by the CoI anchored the cause of the data breach on critical gaps in the perceptions and conceptualization around cybersecurity at SingHealth, as well as the manner of implementation, and practice.

Cybersecurity Basics & Overview of eHealth

The *SingHealth* cyber-attack is one of several high-profile incidents that have made the global healthcare sector a cynosure of negative media attention and much public outcry in recent years. Certain common themes have featured frequently along the trails of these incidents, including poor cybersecurity awareness, unhealthy system and infrastructure security practices, gaps in policy and governance frameworks, and insufficiencies in the conceptualization and understanding of cybersecurity.

These themes highlight a recurring strain of similarities that are altogether indicative of the reality that the pervasiveness and proliferation of various eHealth innovations, systems, and applications in global healthcare, powered by modern information and communications technologies, have created and perpetuated a threat domain. This threat domain is on wherein policy and regulation struggles to keep pace with development, standardization faces several contextual challenges, and technical capacity is largely deficient. The consequences, nonetheless, have remained dire.

Thus, we end up with a soft, high-value target for criminal masterminds, who have continued to scourge the global healthcare sector for financial gain. Class action lawsuits with lingered proceedings, strained financial capacities owing to huge compensation payouts, and the mistrustful sentiments and disrepute that trails emanating debates in many circles. All of these have been the direct impact of this unfortunate convolution.

The 2020 Healthcare Cybersecurity Report[3] by Herjavec Group notes: "more than 93 percent of healthcare organizations have experienced a data breach over the past three years, and 57 percent have had more than five data breaches during the same timeframe". It, therefore, becomes necessary to begin to forge a progressive path towards safer, as well as more secure and trustworthy applications of eHealth in global healthcare.

This chapter introduces cybersecurity as a multi-dimensional concept, with an overview of eHealth and its various applications across domains of modern healthcare, while also discussing healthcare data, as well as the invariants that apply to this unique data class. In addition, the chapter features discussions about user interactions with information and communications technologies (ICTs), as the fulcrum of underlying causes in healthcare cybersecurity incidents.

Cybersecurity as a Concept

Cybersecurity is a composite multi-dimensional concept with many existing definitions. However, the best of these definitions underscore four panels as the aspects that form the objects and focus of a robust approach to conceptualizing cybersecurity. They are *Information Technology Assets* (Infrastructure such as servers, platforms, and networks, as well as systems & devices), *People/Users* (personnel, clients, and vendors), *Processes* (e.g., customer service, sales, purchasing, audits, etc.), and *Policies* (established to govern data, information, network operations, etc.). Figure 1.1 depicts this conceptualization.

Information Technology Assets encompass the Infrastructure, Systems, Platforms, and Devices that feature in an eHealth deployment. These include the servers and platforms (on site and off site / cloud) that host data and services in order to provide the utilities that support operations, the network mediums over which these utilities are provisioned, and the end-point systems and devices that are used to access these utilities, for performing various operations. These systems

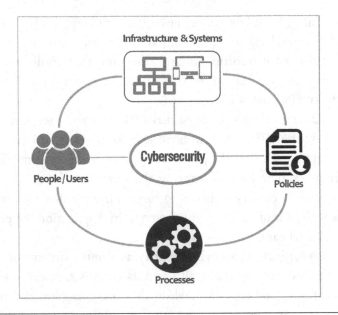

Figure 1.1   Four Panels of Cybersecurity.

and devices could include mobile phones, computers, tablet devices, and other information technology (IT) systems.

People/Users refer to the human agents that interface with Infrastructure for various purposes. They could be personnel who rely on the utilities provided by the Infrastructure to render services, clients who benefit from these rendered services, which sometimes requires them to interface with the Infrastructure directly/indirectly, or vendors who rely on the Infrastructure to provide services to the organization.

Processes refer to various organizational operations that are supported by the services and utilities provided by Infrastructure. They could include a wide range of activities ranging from customer service, to sales, purchasing, audit, and distribution, to mention a few.

Policies are the organization-wide prescriptions that guide and regulate how Infrastructure, People, and Processes function and co-interact around key organizational assets (like data and information). In the most excellent deployments, the design of these prescriptions aligns with wider-acceptable best practices in the industry of business operations.

As a concept, cybersecurity cuts across these Four Panels. Uniting them by a uniform body of procedures and practices, which aims to ensure that all four panels coalesce towards fulfilling the goals and visions of an organization. This is important because, in an increasingly digitized World, the seamless co-interaction and inter-operation of these four Panels in a manner that is secure, reliable, and efficient, may spell the difference between success & failure, profit & liability, progress & bankruptcy for an organization.

Overview & Applications of eHealth

eHealth is an umbrella term that over the last decade has seen growing popularity in the fields of medicine and public health. The World Health Organization broadly defined eHealth as "the use of information and communication technologies (ICT) for health" – a fairly simple and straightforward definition that, however, involves several facets of interactions and supporting technologies coming together to enhance access to quality healthcare, and support service delivery at an affordable cost.

Over the years, eHealth has been seen to involve the deployment of a wide range of information and communication technologies (ICTs) (including mobile telephony, artificial intelligence, voice recognition, speech translation, video conferencing, wired & wireless communication, digital sensing & imaging, computational analytics, bioinformatics / biomedical informatics), supported by electronic devices, for various applications in Healthcare. However, and as illustrated in Figure 1.2, different nomenclatures characterize the coinage of these applications, based on particular utilities, features, and capabilities.

For instance, *mHealth* or *mobile Health* combines the portability of mobile technology with the ubiquity of wireless telecommunications for the delivery of healthcare services. This could be for the purposes of training, awareness & information dissemination, emergency reporting, data collection, or locating healthcare facilities.

Similarly, *TeleHealth* is the provisioning of remote clinical and non-clinical healthcare services over telecommunication channels by leveraging electronic ICTs when service delivery cannot take place physically.

On the one hand, this is applicable for clinical purposes such as medical diagnosis, patient monitoring, physical therapy, off-site surgeries, consultation (between healthcare professionals and patients,

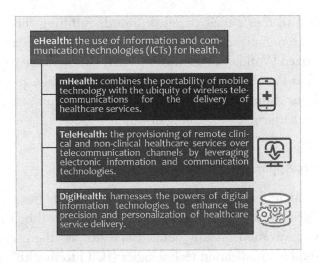

eHealth: the use of information and communication technologies (ICTs) for health.

mHealth: combines the portability of mobile technology with the ubiquity of wireless telecommunications for the delivery of healthcare services.

TeleHealth: the provisioning of remote clinical and non-clinical healthcare services over telecommunication channels by leveraging electronic information and communication technologies.

DigiHealth: harnesses the powers of digital information technologies to enhance the precision and personalization of healthcare service delivery.

Figure 1.2 Overview of eHealth.

and among healthcare professionals), medical reminders & follow-ups, and treatment prescription. While on the other hand, it is also applicable for non-clinical purposes like continuing medical education, and health administration. However, when TeleHealth particularly focuses on clinical healthcare services, it's often been referred to as *TeleMedicine*.

In the same vein, *Digital Health* or *digiHealth* harnesses the powers of digitalization (or digital information technologies) to enhance the precision and personalization of healthcare service delivery. Essentially, it seeks to interconnect data-driven technologies, competences, and capabilities from across multiple domains to improve the effectiveness of healthcare delivery, as well as the general health and wellness of human populations. DigiHealth has been widely applied for clinical decision support, as well as assistive and rehabilitative purposes.

Recent times have seen a wide range of systems and devices feature in the context and operations of eHealth. They include hospital information systems (HIS), mobile phones/smartphones, computers, tablet devices, cyber-physical systems, sensor-based smart wearables (watches, glasses, headgears/headsets, etc.), data-driven decision support systems (DSS), RFID-based implants and ingestibles, robotic scanners, digital imaging devices, personal digital assistants (PDAs), and various forms of patient monitoring devices, among others. These are to mention a few.

eHealth has contributed many benefits to the practice of modern medicine and healthcare delivery, which cannot be overstated. It has helped in bringing quality healthcare to communities that hitherto were unconnected to the global healthcare delivery chain due to impassable road networks, lack of funding, shortage or lack of health-care staff, and language barriers. Several researches have also reported how various applications of eHealth have helped lower the cost of healthcare delivery for both administrators and consumers. It has helped in building confidence in both healthcare staff and patients, and generally helped to strengthen the healthcare systems of entire countries and regions.

Indeed, the quality of healthcare and service delivery shares a strong correlation with the quality and reliability of patient health data that is available to inform healthcare decisions. However, health-care data remains of a rather delicate, private, and confidential nature. This is because the life of the patient or care-receiver depends on its accuracy and consistency in real time, as well as its availability at all times, while the sanctity of their civil liberties could very well depend on its confidentiality.

In many jurisdictions, EHRs (or healthcare data) form an integral part of healthcare delivery, while being fully integrated into national agendas for digitalization and technology development.

Healthcare Data Invariants: Integrity, Confidentiality, and Availability

Today, healthcare data (or EHRs) are worth over $400 USD per patient record[4], while administrative access credentials sell for an average of over $3,000 USD[5] on the global black market. This high value placed on EHRs is traceable, directly or indirectly, to certain well-known invariants that characterize and determine the utilities that EHRs avail for quality healthcare delivery in the era of digitalization. These invariants – Integrity, Confidentiality, and Availability – which probably first emerged in a 1977 Publication on *"Audit and Evaluation of Computer Security"* by the United States Department of Commerce (National Bureau of Standards), have today become very well known, widely applied, and venerable.

Integrity is the characteristic of consistency, completeness, veri-fiability, accuracy, and authenticity throughout the life cycle of a data or information element. Integrity has both physical and logical (non-physical) aspects, and in many cases, these are a function of the practices and realities that originate at the design and developmental phases of data collection, processing, and storage mechanisms, before rippling upwards. Integrity is a key determinant of reliability, as it determines the extent to which data can be trusted as valid enough to be able to inform decisions, reliably.

With respect to EHRs, and indeed other forms of data, Integrity faces a number of risks. This includes human errors that could originate at the point of entry or manipulation, malicious data and system operations and interactions, as well as mismatch errors that could result from moving or replicating data across different storage points. In addition, bugs and misconfigurations could affect concurrency in data (processing) operations, also including malware that seeks to alter and compromise data and information, and system failures that could affect data functions across multiple points. Indeed, to compromise Integrity is to diminish the trustworthiness of data for any purpose, and at all points throughout its life cycle.

Confidentiality relates to the structures of authorization, modes of access, and patterns of use that apply to data elements throughout their life cycle. It is the duty of enforcing the authority to possess/access, so that data does not get into the wrong hands. To succeed in this duty, the prevention of such encounters with data elements that might prove inimical to the interests of data subjects is critical. This is without exceptions to purposes, intent, or actions that might include viewing, sharing/transmitting, usage, or disclosure; and particularly when such an encounter is unintentional, unauthorized, unlawful, unnecessary, or unscrupulous.

There exists a number of risks to the Confidentiality of healthcare data. These include stolen or compromised access credentials, escalated privilege levels, misconfigured or poorly secured systems and devices for storing, processing, or manipulating data, open transmission over public analogue or digital media, disposal techniques that are not resilient against recovery and reconstruction, and existing vulnerabilities in acquired database systems and infrastructure. In many contexts, to compromise confidentiality is to undermine the legitimate claims to the privacy of data subjects in ways that oppose the wider-acceptable prescriptions and norms regarding digital and civil rights.

Availability pertains to the guarantee that data elements and the information they translate into are always and promptly accessible at all times, at all such points, and for all such uses, functions, and operations that are authorized, ethical, and lawful – in order to preserve the utility of data and information, regardless of prevailing realities. In many cases, this guarantee has less to do with the actual data and information elements themselves, and more to do with the status of the devices, infrastructure, systems, and networks that avail these data and information.

Perhaps one of the most popular risks to Availability is having more concurrent usage of digital utilities than overall computing resources are able to cater for, effectively and efficiently. This could result from non-malicious factors such as periods of high service demand that see many users seeking access to the digital services that an organization provides – a phenomenon technically referred to as *"Flash Crowds"*. It could also be the outcome of malicious attempts to overwhelm computing resources in order to hinder legitimate use – a phenomenon known as a *"Denial of Service (DoS)"* attack; or a *"Distributed Denial of Service (DDoS)"* attack (when it involves enlisting the capacity of other hijacked / compromised machines to amplify the impact of the attack).

However, it is possible to endanger Availability through incidents that result in data corruption, disconnection/inaccessibility, or erasure, which might result from malware activities, system/network malfunction and failure, or human actions like disconnecting or disabling system and network connections. In essence, however, to compromise the availability of healthcare data is to grind to a halt all such uses, functions, and operations that rely on the information that such healthcare data provides, whether as part of products or services.

Figure 1.3 illustrates the triadic relationship between Confidentiality, Availability, and Integrity when it comes to Healthcare Data (or EHRs).

Generally, these three Invariants also incorporate imperatives for ensuring their quality and security. However, these imperatives are usually also a function of the standards and rules adopted by existing and binding frameworks for governing and regulating data functions, operations, and interactions from a higher level. In jurisdictions that consider healthcare data and information essential for the preservation and functioning of society, these Invariants are ostensibly the reason

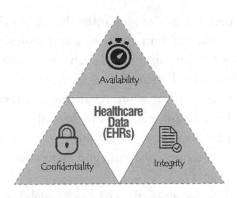

Figure 1.3   Healthcare Data (EHRs) Invariants.

for classifying the devices, infrastructure, systems, and networks that avail these data and information, as "critical infrastructure".

Anytime there is a compromise of the invariants of *Integrity*, *Confidentiality*, and/or *Availability*, the saying in lay terms often follows – "data has been breached". Although, many times, the use of this phrase may neither correctly, nor entirely reflect the true situation of a data incident in reality. However, the phrase generally describes the idea that a malicious (and often external) attack against a data invariant has turned out successful. In reality, however, data incidents may not necessarily be a handiwork of malicious entities attacking from the outside only. It could also be the result of a naive (possibly inadvertent), or malicious (usually intentional) insider action or operation; or a system failure/malfunction, in which case it could more correctly be referred to as a "leakage".

It is also important to note that within the domain of healthcare, the *Confidentiality* of data is often the most attacked of all three invariants, since it tends to bring the most direct financial reward to the attackers upon success. Attacks against *Availability* and *Integrity* more often aim to cause reputational damage and loss of revenue, or coerce healthcare facilities and service providers into paying certain amounts of money to reverse or remedy the impact of such situations.

Healthcare Information & Communication Technology and People

The healthcare sector is one in which ICTs and people frequently interface and interact for various purposes that pertain to healthcare service delivery. These people could include non-technical users like patients, patient caregivers, doctors/physicians, nurses, pharmacists, third-party vendors, public health professionals, social workers, volunteers, and visitors to healthcare facilities, technical users like system and network administrators, and IT support personnel, to mention a few, as well as other support staff like cleaners/janitors, doorkeepers, and guards.

Some of these individuals harness the utilities and capabilities of healthcare ICTs (otherwise known as eHealth) to perform and support various uses, functions, and operations that coalesce towards improving the quality of healthcare service delivery. Others help to maintain and support these healthcare ICTs in order to ensure that they are performing securely, optimally, and productively. Yet others work to ensure that the environments where these healthcare ICTs are domiciled remain ideally safe, healthful, and comfortable.

Unfortunately, however, these people/user groups, the majority of whom are often technically untrained in the discourse of cybersecurity have frequently posed the most formidable fault lines to eHealth cybersecurity.

Several independent reports (including by Russian cybersecurity giant, Kaspersky[6]) estimate that about half (47–52%) of the organizational cybersecurity incidents that occur annually, particularly as pertains to data, have origins that can be directly or indirectly traced to various user actions and operations, even within the global healthcare sector.

These various groups of users have often presented the human lapses through which cybercriminals have continued to scourge the global healthcare sector. In some cases, these criminal operations have been abetted (even unwittingly) by human actions of naiveness, inadvertency, unawareness, disinterestedness, unscrupulousness, and recklessness; while in other cases, they have been catalysed by innate human feelings and emotions of desperation, love, altruism, nonchalance, hatred, disgruntlement, malice, avarice, and discontent. This framework of actions and sentiments generally increases the susceptibility of these user groups to maliciously intended schemes and strategies, making them the metaphorical "weak links" in many cybersecurity chains.

On some occasions, the devices that they bring with them to participate in the digital spaces around healthcare facilities have unknowingly participated in cybersecurity incidents. These digital spaces could be those that either enable remote work or support on-site work. However, when these devices – which could be poorly secured, not well-configured, shared devices, or laced with malware – connect to digital spaces that are otherwise secure, they carry across this framework of vulnerabilities and apparently undermine the security status of these digital spaces. At other times, these security weaknesses devolve from gaps and inadequacies in the abilities of support staff to effectively discern and stall potential cybersecurity threats and risks before they result in actual security incidents.

Even then, the shifting nature of human behaviour further adds another level of difficulty to the discourse around Users and the security of ICTs. Where it is possible to model human behaviour across multiple security contexts and situations, consistently and accurately, then algorithmic approaches are easily deployable to meet the challenges of human vulnerability when it comes to cybersecurity, even effectively. However, this often poses a problem that is not only complex, but also complicated. Since behaviours are basically a manifestation of complex strains of sentiments and undertones embedded in the psychology and emotions of users, which are often difficult to spot and completely rehabilitate, even more difficult to circumspect exhaustively, and sometimes impossible to exorcise permanently.

For example, a network administrator attempting to deploy a network service quickly might, in a bid to multi-task and enhance productivity, apply a shell script to automatically configure and host the service on the organization's network. Sometimes, this administrator might omit to take cognisance of certain default configuration parameters that do not meet the security standards, policies, and operational frameworks of the organization. Similarly, a user trying to access their online social networks using the office Internet connection that is only accessible on corporate devices might attempt to upload multimedia (pictures and videos) by plugging in a personal removable device. Failing to consider that malware could infiltrate the corporate network through this means.

In addition, the doorkeeper to a healthcare facility might not understand the risks to cybersecurity posed by an inability to present a valid access card at all points of entry (regardless of the associated circumstance or the person involved). Hence, this individual might manually override or subvert access validation protocols for a person in a wheelchair who is unable to reach high enough to swipe their access card. An elderly visitor who is struggling to drag along several bags is also likely to be granted the same compromise; even an employee who seems unable to find their access card at the time. Such a doorkeeper might be apparently oblivious of the fact that these incidents could well be forerunners or precursors in action, as part of a coordinated security violation strategy.

In the same way, a janitor or cleaner might not understand the cybersecurity risks posed by the unavailability of a critical system, network service, or connection. As a result, he could accidentally trip over a network or power cable in the course of their cleaning duties, and then casually ignore the necessity of immediately calling the attention of the technical IT staff to the incident. Eventually, this may result in disruptions to service availability and delivery to the lower legs of the network from that point of connection down the line; or even result in disruptions to the effectiveness of services rendered by the systems and devices that depend on that particular connection remaining online.

In summary, it is the holy grail of eHealth cybersecurity, and perhaps cybersecurity generally, to essentially protect and safeguard the sanctity of the three Invariants of Confidentiality, Integrity, and Availability. In practice, however, this is often only achievable by deploying a multi-dimensional approach that factors in the various interactions between Infrastructure & Systems, the People (technical and non-technical Users, as well as support staff) that interface with them, the business Processes that rely on them, and the organizational Policies that provide the governance framework for all of these.

Notes

1 Choo, C. (2019, January 09). *SingHealth cyber attack a result of human lapses, IT system weaknesses: COI report*. Today. https://www.todayonline.com/singapore/singhealth-cyber-attack-result-human-lapses-it-system-weaknesses-coi-report

2 Singapore Ministry of Communications and Information (2019, January 10). *Public Report of the Committee of Inquiry (CoI) into the cyber-attack on Singapore Health Services Private Limited Patient Database*. https://www.mci.gov.sg/pressroom/news-and-stories/pressroom/2019/1/public-report-of-the-coi

3 Herjavec Group (2020). The 2020 Healthcare Cybersecurity Report: A Special Report from the Editors at Cybersecurity Ventures. https://www.herjavecgroup.com/wp-content/uploads/2019/12/Healthcare-Cybersecurity-Report-2020.pdf

4 Davis, J. (2019, July 23). Data Breaches Cost Healthcare $6.5M, or $429 per Patient Record. *Health IT Security*. https://healthitsecurity.com/news/data-breaches-cost-healthcare-6.5m-or-429-per-patient-record

5 Digital Shadows Photon Research Team (2020). *From Exposure to Takeover: The 15 billion stolen credentials allowing account takeover*. Digital Shadows. https://resources.digitalshadows.com/whitepapers-and-reports/from-exposure-to-takeover

6 Kaspersky (n.d.). The Human Factor in IT Security: How Employees are Making Businesses Vulnerable from Within. *Kaspersky Daily*. https://www.kaspersky.com/blog/the-human-factor-in-it-security/

2

THE CYBERSECURITY THREAT LANDSCAPE FOR eHEALTH

Introduction

While it is true that cybersecurity risks are able to ripple through the entire digital apparatuses of healthcare organizations, they often originate and spread from within particular ecosystems of operations and interactions within the business of healthcare. Hence, it is important for professionals and administrators alike to be able to answer certain critical questions at the point of adding new digital models and operations to existing corporate repertoires.

What (new) ecosystem(s) of digital interactions does this new scope of healthcare service or operation created (or expand)? What elements participate in this new ecosystem(s)? In order to safeguard operations effectively within this new healthcare digital ecosystem(s), what are the dimensions of cybersecurity to consider? The answers to these questions are crucial in order to ensure that new business models and operations do not exacerbate existing cybersecurity risks, amplify the effect of vulnerabilities, and extend the scope of impact for cyber threats and attacks in healthcare organizations. However, to answer these questions effectively, a robust understanding of the threat landscape is indispensable, especially knowing that the cybersecurity threat landscape continues to shift and metamorphose frequently and rapidly within very short periods.

For instance, in the aftermath of the COVID-19 Pandemic (year 2020), many healthcare organizations were forced to implement a rapid digital transition, including migrating operations to new platforms and environments in the "cloud". The aim was to help them cope with the imperatives for physical distancing in a way that does not upturn their entire chain of operations. In the process, there was the creation of new digital ecosystems around existing business repertoires. However, for many of these instances, it also meant a significant change in the usual cybersecurity threat landscape for the organizations involved[1]. The healthcare sector was among the first hit by the wave of cyber-attacks reported in the early days of the lockdowns occasioned by the Pandemic.

As many hospitals and healthcare facilities turned to eHealth in a bid to limit physical interface with non-COVID-19 patients, and manage the limited stocks and supplies of personal protective equipment to cater to the critically ill and hospitalized patients, new remote capabilities opened up a metamorphosed threat landscape that created new opportunities for cybercriminals. There was the amplification of well-known malicious techniques, even as new strategies for exploitation emerged. As a result, the statistics on cyber incidents and attacks to the healthcare sector exceeded, within a few short months, the figures reported over the last few years as annual statistics.

Within the first month of the Pandemic-occasioned lockdowns alone, several independent reports (including by American-Israeli IT security giant, Check Point[2]) revealed that cybersecurity incidents had more than doubled the figures reported over the previous few years. Insights from Spanish cybersecurity company – Panda Security[3], also revealed that more of the targeted organizations were in the global healthcare sector (including the World Health Organization[4]). Thus, it is important to re-present and discuss the cybersecurity threat landscape, particularly as it pertains to the global healthcare sector. This would help enhance a better understanding of the status and realities of this threat landscape, and ultimately build capacity for robust, coordinated, and effective bottom-up response strategies to the cybersecurity threats that trail the various applications of ICTs in healthcare.

Thus, this chapter presents and traverses the Cybersecurity Threat Landscape for eHealth, and then discusses an overview of what happens when cybersecurity incidents target the healthcare sector. It further presents the more common threats to users, threats to systems & devices, threats to infrastructure, threats to processes/operations, and threats to policies that feature in this Threat Landscape. It then goes on to highlight and elucidate a repertoire of risk factors that help to insure the success of malicious activities that target the healthcare sector.

The Cybersecurity Threat Landscape for eHealth

Although not very different from the general cybersecurity threat landscape *per se*, the particular high-value nature of the assets that feature in the global healthcare sector (including user data and critical infrastructure) make these assets the priced trophies that criminal masterminds crave to lay hands on. This is probably the reason why healthcare cybersecurity incidents are relatively more popular and high profile.

By deploying an array of tools, techniques, and strategies, all varied in their sophistication, attackers seem to retain the upper hand as preparedness and response efforts struggle to keep pace with the dynamic nature of the cybersecurity threat landscape. Indeed, threats to cybersecurity in Healthcare have been discovered to pertain to end users; the applications that avail various healthcare functions and services; and the systems and devices that are used to access these user applications. While at the same time, also targeting the data that they generate, store, process, and use; the infrastructure that underlies and powers these systems and applications, and the information that are transmitted over these infrastructures; the business processes and operations that rely on the efficient functioning of these Infrastructures; and the policies that define and guide interactions within this realm.

Therefore, it is useful, and perhaps intuitive to consider a layered approach to understanding the Cybersecurity Threat Landscape to eHealth. Figure 2.1 presents a layered conceptualization of this Threat Landscape. Indeed, what is (or should be) the goal of cybersecurity

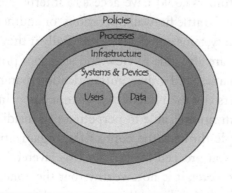

Figure 2.1 A Layered Approach to Understanding the eHealth Cybersecurity Threat Landscape.

for eHealth is to protect Users and their Data from malicious actors. In order for this to be effectively pursued, Systems (hardware and software) and Devices, which have the most direct impact and interface with users and data, need to be protected. In the same way, this applies to the Infrastructure that provides the framework for interactions, which systems and devices often leverage to interface with users and their data. The processes and operations that necessitate these interactions between systems & devices on the one hand, and then users & data on the other hand, over corporate infrastructure are also critical considerations in this Threat Landscape. While at the same time not neglecting the policies and procedures that define the context for these various facets of interactions.

Therefore, within this eHealth Threat Landscape, policies and procedures should clearly define what users and data participate in particular processes and operations, the systems and devices permitted to feature in these interactions, as well as the infrastructural provisions necessary to power these interactions. This is because gaps in the policy are capable of endangering processes and operations, and, by extension, putting infrastructure at risk, thereby jeopardizing the security of interactions involving medical systems & devices, as well as users and their healthcare data.

Here is a way to look at it. When healthcare organizational policies fail to define clearly the operations of customer service, particularly in terms of boundaries and limits, it may seem right to some employees to bring clients/customers beyond the general waiting area/reception of the facility into their personal workspaces. Within this private space, these customers could have access to internal network connections and be able to rattle firewall operations, or enumerate and reconnoitre healthcare systems and devices, especially if they have malicious intentions. They are also able to view and snapshot private user interfaces, see usernames and other authentication parameters, thereby endangering users and their data. In essence, a policy insufficiency of a healthcare organization is able to perpetuate an insidious susceptibility that can ripple through the core of the organization's assets. The same is true as you proceed inwards in this layered threat landscape (Figure 2.1). However, it is noteworthy that the conceptualization in Figure 2.1 is merely idealistic. Because, in reality, corporate arrangements may not particularly reflect this exact representation.

While it is often commonplace to use the terms *"threat"* and *"attack"* synonymously or analogously when referring to happenings in cybersecurity, even in the context of healthcare, they do not actually mean the same thing, at least not technically. The fundamental difference generally lies in the notions of *"intention"* and *"intentionality"*. Whereas "intention" is a function of the purpose/motive/aim/goal, "intentionality" is a function of the process/manner/method.

A threat is an insidious security condition, the creation of which may or may not have been intentional and features intention that may or may not be malicious. However, its behaviour and action could, nonetheless, enable or directly result in a security violation. An attack, on the other hand, is a security violation that intentionally compromises a security condition, typically with malicious intentions.

Another concept that often features in this context is the concept of *"vulnerability"*. A vulnerability is a security gap, susceptibility, or weakness that a threat takes advantage of, in order to result in a security violation. So, in other words, and in many instances, threats must meet vulnerabilities, in order for security to be successfully compromised, or attacks orchestrated. Figure 2.2 depicts this relationship.

Vulnerabilities, in this case, could exist in users (their behaviours, propensities, and activities); infrastructure, systems & devices (by virtue of their design, operations, and usage); processes & operations (concerning their security resilience), as well as policies (in terms of their robustness). In essence, Vulnerabilities are often a product of inherent lapses in the systems, devices, strategies, processes, and procedures put in place for security, protection, and defence.

For example, a weak/unchanged default user password is a Vulnerability. Writing it on a sticky note and pasting it close to a computer in order not to forget it, that is a Threat. When a third party

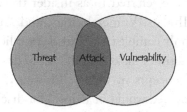

Figure 2.2   Threat, Vulnerability, and Attack.

leverages this condition to gain unauthorized access to a user account on an eHealth product or service, a security violation has occurred.

Similarly, a healthcare computer system without anti-malware installed poses a Vulnerability. Removable devices that connect to such a computer are Threats. However, when a piece of malware successfully transloads from these removable devices onto the computer, a security violation has occurred. Realize that this violation could be an unwitting outcome of the Threat action. It could also represent the success of a deliberate attempt to infiltrate the computer system with malicious intention, in which case referring to it as an attack would be right.

In the same vein, a misconfigured medical system or database server poses a Threat. An inexperienced systems administrator or organizational policies that allow users to configure and reconfigure corporate devices arbitrarily – these are pre-disposing Vulnerabilities to this Threat. A healthcare data leak is a security violation that could result from this situation, even though no malicious intentions may have been associated with it.

In addition, a healthcare organizational policy that allows employees more privileged access to data and information resources than is ordinarily needed for their job functions is a Vulnerability. Such an employee in this role becomes a Threat. However, to use this privilege to siphon sensitive data or information maliciously for personal financial gain is an attack that violates security.

Again, an open Wi-Fi connection without an authentication access code at a healthcare facility is a Vulnerability. An outsider who connects to this resource without an authorization becomes a Threat. When such an outsider undertakes a malicious action under this condition, an Attack has taken place.

Notice also that Threats could have origins that are either internal (in which case they are referred to as insider threats) or external. In practice, however, Threats, Vulnerabilities, and Attacks share a relationship that is not only complex but is also complicated. The nature of this relationship sometimes makes it difficult to draw a distinct demarcation along these concepts in theory. However, understanding the descriptions here provided would be helpful for discerning the contemporary realities of the Cybersecurity Threat Landscape for eHealth.

Threat Agents to Cybersecurity of eHealth

Threats exist or manifest when Threat Agents exploit, attempt to exploit, or perpetuate a vulnerability. Thus, these Threat Agents are an indispensable factor in the discourse around cybersecurity in eHealth. Indeed, the eHealth Cybersecurity Threat Landscape is one that has continued to feature different players. Threat Agents that have featured in this Landscape include individual entities, independent groups, corporate entities, sovereign (nation-state) entities, or non-sovereign (but sovereign-sponsored) entities. In other words, basically, Threat Agents to eHealth cybersecurity include individual and non-individual entities, which could be either independent or sovereign-affiliated, as well as sovereign entities.

Individual Entities could be hackers who have technical skills in the workings and operations of computer/information security. They could also include malicious individuals who might not have technical skills but may seek to undertake malicious operations through non-technical means. Then, they could also be naive human actors (internal or external) without malicious intent, but whose unwitting actions and activities could be no less inimical to security interests and goals.

Independent Groups are associations of malicious individual entities united by a common vision or mission that could be political, ideological, cultural, financial, patriotic, or otherwise. As part of their repertoire of operations, they could feature certain levels of technical competence. Whereas, the inspiration behind their operations could be terror/insurrection, propaganda, extremism, activism, or wild enthusiasm.

In some cases, sovereign governments seeking to undertake malicious cyber operations for various reasons could sponsor Individuals and Independent Groups. In this capacity, they qualify as **Sovereign-sponsored/Sovereign-affiliated Threat Agents**.

Corporate Entities with competing or partnering interests could also pose as threat agents to eHealth cybersecurity. When competing interest is involved, malicious intentions usually feature with the aim of sabotaging corporate interests or the reputation of the target organization. However, when partnering interests are involved, actions of inadvertence could equally create or perpetuate threat situations that might be inimical to corporate security interests. Compared to

Individual Entities and Independent Groups that are not sovereign-sponsored, Corporate Threat Entities with malicious intentions often feature more threat resource capabilities.

Threat resource capabilities in this regard could be financial, technical (in terms of capacity of skillset and toolset), and/or infrastructural.

Sovereign Entities are nation states that undertake malicious cyber operations in order to safeguard or assert national interests that could be political, trade-related, reputational, or security-related. Nation-state entities are usually able to deploy a seemingly infinite amount of threat resource capabilities to insure and amplify the impact of their threat-attack operations.

It is not commonplace for sovereign and sovereign-sponsored/sovereign-affiliated entities to threaten cybersecurity in the context of healthcare. At the same time, it is not impossible. Since financial benefit is known to be a primary motivation behind a vast majority (over 80%[5]) of cybersecurity incidents (data breaches), even in the healthcare sector, it is quite rare that nation-states and nation-state-sponsored entities would target healthcare institutions with this goal in mind.

However, there are uncommon cases where healthcare organizations, their systems, and infrastructure provide a window or leeway into the operations and activities of bigger targets of interest (such as national governments, or the armed forces). There are also more common cases where healthcare facilities hold electronic health records of influential individuals that are of national or international interest. In such cases, healthcare organizations could become targets of sovereign and sovereign-sponsored/sovereign-affiliated entities on the path to pursuing these larger interests.

For instance, multiple sources in the aftermath of the 2018 *SingHealth* cyber-attack (such as the *UK Telegraph*[6]) reported allegations that the attack might have been a targeted state-coordinated, or state-sponsored incident that sought to lay hands on the electronic health records of influential individuals in the Singaporean government at the time, including the Prime Minister – Lee Hsien Loong.

Cybersecurity Incidents in Healthcare

When cybersecurity incidents happen in healthcare due to the malicious or inadvertent actions/activities of threat agents, certain

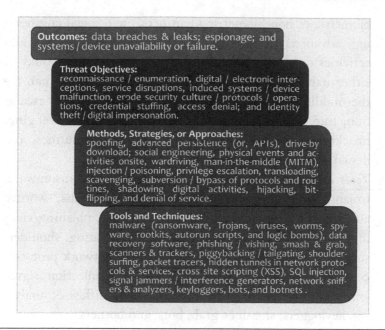

Outcomes: data breaches & leaks; espionage; and systems / device unavailability or failure.

Threat Objectives:
reconnaissance / enumeration, digital / electronic interceptions, service disruptions, induced systems / device malfunction, erode security culture / protocols / operations, credential stuffing, access denial; and identity theft / digital impersonation.

Methods, Strategies, or Approaches:
spoofing, advanced persistence (or, APIs), drive-by download; social engineering, physical events and activities onsite, wardriving, man-in-the-middle (MITM), injection / poisoning, privilege escalation, transloading, scavenging, subversion / bypass of protocols and routines, shadowing digital activities, hijacking, bit-flipping, and denial of service.

Tools and Techniques:
malware (ransomware, Trojans, viruses, worms, spyware, rootkits, autorun scripts, and logic bombs), data recovery software, phishing / vishing, smash & grab, scanners & trackers, piggybacking / tailgating, shoulder-surfing, packet tracers, hidden tunnels in network protocols & services, cross site scripting (XSS), SQL injection, signal jammers / interference generators, network sniffers & analyzers, keyloggers, bots, and botnets .

Figure 2.3   When Healthcare Cybersecurity Incidents Happen.

outcomes usually manifest, and several tools and techniques, methods or strategies, as well as threat objectives frequently feature as part of the threat-attack processes and operations that lead to these outcomes (Figure 2.3).

Typically, these **Outcomes** include *data breaches & leaks, espionage,* and *unavailability or failure of medical and healthcare IT systems/devices.* Espionage, however, is seldom an outcome when cybersecurity incidents target healthcare facilities, except, as previously highlighted, in cases where the systems or infrastructure of a healthcare organization provides a window/leeway into the operations and activities of a bigger entity of interest, such as the government or armed forces.

The trail that leads towards these outcomes features:

- **Threat Objectives** such as reconnaissance/enumeration, digital/electronic interceptions, service disruptions, induced systems/device malfunction, erode security culture/protocols/ operations, credential stuffing, and identity theft/digital impersonation;
- **Methods, Strategies, or Approaches** like spoofing (of emails, packets, location, addresses, protocol operations, websites,

biometric & non-biometric identifiers, etc.), social engineering, advanced persistence (or, APTs), physical events and activities on site (including insider operations that could be either naive or maliciously intended), wardriving, man-in-the-middle (MITM), injection/poisoning, privilege escalation, transloading, shadowing digital activities, scavenging, hijacking, subversion/bypass of protocols and routines, and denial of service (DoS); and,

- *Tools and Techniques* that include malware (ransomware, trojans, viruses, spyware, rootkits, logic bombs, worms, and autorun scripts), data recovery software, phishing/vishing, scanners & trackers, piggybacking/tailgating, shoulder-surfing, packet tracers, hidden tunnels in network protocols & services, cross-site scripting (XSS), SQL injection, signal jammers/interference generators, network sniffers & analysers, keyloggers, smash & grab, bots, and botnets.

In practice, tools and techniques are integrated as part of methods/strategies/approaches, which are incorporated within the framework of Threat objectives that are geared towards outcomes that become known as cybersecurity incidents. In practice, however, it has been seen that multiple threat objectives can incorporate different methods/strategies/approaches, which, in turn, enlist a wide range of sophisticated tools and techniques (particularly when malicious intentions are involved) in order to bring about cybersecurity incidents.

For instance, as part of a threat-attack objective that aims to cause a medical system failure, an induced malfunction might begin the chain through a privilege escalation that integrates a spoofing technique seeking to impersonate an authorized digital identity in the eyes of the system; before trans-loading a malware or executing an SQL injection on the system or device. Similarly, a threat-attack strategy that seeks to breach electronic health records for financial gain could enlist hardware- or software-based network sniffers and packet analysers in a technique that features physical events on site at the healthcare facility to capture sensitive information (e.g., access credentials), as part of a coordinated digital interception strategy that integrates insider operations.

Pertaining People/Users

People/Users are frequent targets in the cybersecurity threat landscape for healthcare. As discussed in Chapter One, this is because they often pose soft targets for the high-value assets that feature in the global healthcare sector. Sometimes, threats to users could arise from the conscious actions and inadvertencies of other users in the same process/operations chain. Other times, they could be targeted attempts by malicious outsiders to exploit deduced, perceived, or disclosed vulnerabilities for financial gain.

Generally, however, when threats and attacks target people/users in the healthcare sector, they often gun for sensitive *Data* about them, and the *Access Credentials* that they hold. Perhaps, and yet the most common and popular avenue by which these threats/attacks have been known to infiltrate and propagate is through social engineering.

Social Engineering enlists a number of approaches in a practice that aims at conning/manipulating individuals into doing things that they are unlikely to do, given different circumstances. This could include divulging sensitive information, performing actions that are inimical to security interests and goals, or granting otherwise unpermitted concessions.

Social Engineering typically seeks to exploit cognitive biases (sometimes referred to as "bugs in the human hardware"), as well as other psychological and behavioural tendencies/susceptibilities. It is a potent technique because these biases often underlie and inform the most obvious behaviours and actions of users, making them susceptible to certain kinds of external influence by malicious actors. Through Social Engineering, it has proven possible to trick people/users within the healthcare space into divulging sensitive financial details, and account credentials successfully. It is also possible to manipulate or lure them into clicking links or connecting removable devices that ultimately transload and install malicious software, which gave attackers persistent and privileged access to system resources.

Phishing and Vishing are common approaches to social engineering that have often featured in threat-attack situations that target people/users in healthcare. It is an act of impersonating a trusted entity in an electronic communication, in order to obtain sensitive data or information by trick. When this act is perpetrated over an electronic communication that is voice-based (such as a phone call or voice recording), it is referred to as Vishing. However, when it is perpetrated over a text-based communication (like email, chat/instant message, or short message), it is referred to as Phishing.

Other approaches to social engineering include piggybacking or tailgating – a practice of surreptitiously tagging close to someone that has authorized access to a secure or restricted healthcare application/ facility/area, in order to get past a required security check or access validation protocol, and gain access without going through the authorization routines. Also, there is the technique of shoulder-surfing that is applied to observe and possibly memorize security credentials like usernames, passwords, PIN codes, credit card details, and secure URLs by peeping or snooping over shoulders of users at the point of entering these credentials.

In addition, Social Engineering particularly targets people/users in healthcare based information about their schedules, employers, work environment & cultures, online and offline interactions, digital devices and their usage, network connections, and user interfaces & applications. This could be deduced passively (without direct interactions or interface with the targeted users, but rather through publicly accessible sources) or actively (involving direct interactions and interface with users). The preference for social engineering by malicious actors is, perhaps, owing to the fact that it requires almost no technical expertise, and often presents a path of least resistance.

Think about it this way. Why would a malicious individual seeking to gain access to sensitive and high-value healthcare data spend so much time engineering a sophisticated malware as part of a robust attack regimen to breach highly secure organizational servers and systems? When alternatively, they could simply:

- Disguise as a technical staff of the healthcare organization over a phone call to deceive a naive employee with authorized access into divulging login credentials;
- Loiter around a private workspace within the healthcare facility, waiting for a user to step away from their workstation without completely logging off, and then jumping on to continue access using the user's credentials;

- Manipulate a disgruntled technical staff at a hospital, who has authorized access and probably does not know the actual worth of such data on the black market, into transferring such data for a paltry sum;
- Tailgate an employee with authorized access to an otherwise secure healthcare facility that houses electronic health records during peak entry hours on a busy workday, and then implant devices that would enable remote access and siphoning of sensitive data;
- Exploit a trusted relationship or an altruistic tendency of an authorized hospital employee to request use of a personal or work device, and then implant a keylogger or other malware on the device in the process;
- Create an identical replica of a public-facing user interface in order to con an unaware authorized user or employee into providing access credentials; or
- Deduce layouts and content of non-public-facing user interfaces through publicly posted pictures by an unscrupulous user/healthcare professional that shows computer screens; and then create an identical replica to launch a large-scale identity theft targeting employees of a healthcare organization.

The options are indeed numerous, and they all present effective pathways for success, even with little technical expertise. At scale, successful identity theft operations that target a particular healthcare organization can provide very potent advantage for a later credential stuffing cyber-attack, which deploys these stolen identities to automate user login requests across multiple servers or web services using freely available web automation tools and applications. These could be useful foundations for data breaches/leaks, and other forms of healthcare cyber incidents.

However, malicious actors that target people/users could also decide to shadow their digital interactions or electronic communications in order to steal data about them as well as their access credentials. Shadowing in this regard is achievable using Keyloggers – a hardware or software device that is able to trap and record input keystrokes and mouse clicks on digital electronic devices and machines, which are then transmitted to a designated location for the use of the attacker.

Indeed, threats that target healthcare users are latent threats to medical systems and devices, organizational infrastructure, healthcare processes and operations, as well as corporate policies.

Pertaining Systems & Devices

Medical devices and other information and communication technologies (ICTs) used in healthcare often pose an easy target for malicious actors, and for many reasons. This is because security resilience is often times lacking in many of these devices, particularly as they often feature software and hardware that have long been outdated.

Generally, threats and attacks to medical ICT systems and devices target the *Data* and *Information* that they collect, process, access, and store about users (employees, clients, and vendors), and business operations. These threats and attacks usually explore methods and strategies like spoofing, scavenging, injection/poisoning, transloading, hijacking, bit-flipping attacks, and privilege escalation.

These methods and strategies lean towards objectives such as reconnaissance/enumeration, identity theft/digital impersonation, induced malfunction in systems/device, access denial through lockouts and service truncation, and altering data & information. In many cases, by the time these systems and devices come under threat by malicious actors, people and users have long been at risk, with the possibility of having one or more these already compromised.

In spoofing, digital identities are stolen or falsified. The goal being to accrue to an unknown and illegitimate party the otherwise legitimate advantages and benefits accorded to a trusted digital player. The digital identities that could be spoofed in this case range from emails, to data packets, location information, device (physical) addresses, protocol operations, websites, as well as biometric & non-biometric identifiers, to mention a few. A spoofed hospital website or server address could successfully impersonate and pose to users as a legitimate digital actor, in order to obtain their access credentials, data, or other legitimate information. Similarly, a spoofed device address with administrative privileges can pose a legitimate request for users' healthcare data or information domiciled on a secure server.

Scavenging is the practice of searching through physical or logical residues for sensitive information that could be useful for malicious purposes. When scavenging takes place physically, it often happens around a healthcare organization's dumpsites or garbage collection point(s), but when it happens logically, it involves scouring through system log files and error reports for sensitive information that could offer an advantage in a malicious scheme. Data and information that was contained in a casually disposed storage device can also be recovered and reconstructed substantially (and in some cases, completely) using software that is freely available on the Internet, even though the storage device may have been properly formatted or erased prior to disposal. In the same way, sensitive information on printed materials that are casually disposed have also provided an advantage for criminal scavengers.

Similarly, Privilege Escalation seeks to take advantage of a design flaw in a healthcare system or software, in order to gain access to usually protected resources (sensitive data and information) that are otherwise inaccessible to particular users, user groups, or applications. When malicious actors succeed in escalating privilege, it becomes much easier for them to cover their tracks properly by tampering with system/event activity logs. Thereby making it difficult to promptly detect healthcare cybersecurity incidents and respond in a timely and effective manner.

Bit-flipping attacks provide a non-cryptanalytic way for attackers to compromise cryptographic cipher implementations by changing bits in the encrypted information (known as the cipher text) in a way that could bring about a predictable change in the original message. While this attack does not necessarily provide a way for the attackers to learn the content of the original message precisely, it does make it possible to compromise the integrity of particular messages or blocks of messages that rely on a particular cipher channel. In cases where such a cipher channel is required for authentication purposes, a bit-flipping attack could result in a denial of access.

Injection/Poisoning, however, is the practice of introducing or feeding bad/bogus commands and parameters into request or commit operations, in a bid to cause healthcare systems and devices to fail-open and release sensitive user/client data and information that they hold. XSS (cross-site scripts), malicious query statements in SQL (structured query language), packet header, and routing table poisoning; these are common techniques that have been adopted as part of the injection/poisoning threat-attack regimen.

In addition, malicious actors could seek to hijack systems and devices belonging to users and their employers/healthcare organizations, in order to gain remote control over these machines as avenues for amplifying the strength and impact of subsequent malicious schemes. Under this form of coordinated control, these compromised machines remain subject to the whims and caprices of the malicious actors, who are able to instruct them to carry out a broad range of malicious activities in order to remove attention from the persons of the real attackers. Such machines become "zombies" under the influence of the attacker.

Alternatively, malicious threat actors could explore avenues for directly or indirectly transloading malware onto medical ICT systems and devices for the purpose of disrupting normal system and device functions/operations, as well as denying access. Malware has been a common tool often featuring in the threat-attack processes that target medical systems and devices. A portmanteau term that integrates "malicious + software", malware exists in various types/kinds, namely, spyware, ransomware, Trojans, viruses, rootkits, logic bombs, worms, and automated running (Autorun) scripts.

There are deeper technical characteristics that help to distinguish more clearly between these various sorts of malware. However, in the most basic sense, worms and viruses differ in that worms are autonomous self-replicating malware, while viruses replicate by binding to relevant user files and are generally under the control of an external influence that is usually the attacker or malware author. On the other hand, Trojans often come disguised as software that is legitimate and harmless (like games, software, etc.), while ransomware operate by hijacking and denying access to systems/devices and the data that they hold, until a fee (known as the ransom) is paid.

Similarly, spyware covertly transmits data and information about a computer's operations and activities to an external malicious actor, while rootkits enable background/backdoor access to systems, devices, and user applications, and then masking its existence and operations in order to evade detection. In the same way, logic bombs are malware built into application software to activate certain malicious behaviours when particular logical conditions are satisfied. Whereas, autorun scripts are malicious codes that activate automatically as soon as they interface with systems & devices, making them able to bypass regular security checks.

The capacity of malware to orchestrate colossal damage and wreak sheer havoc to eHealth services and healthcare operations is quite well established. They are able to add false information and markers to patients' scans and imaging reports in order to misinform medical diagnosis and compromise the integrity of healthcare services. In addition, they can automatically dump, or siphon sensitive personal healthcare-related information in massive volumes; tamper with readings of medical monitoring devices; and alter doses in medication delivered through electronic infusion pumps & valves. Malware are also able to surreptitiously download other malicious components (through a strategy known as drive-by); and give malicious external actors a sustained foothold on the digital operations of healthcare facilities. Indeed, the menacing impact of malware on the global healthcare sector is a danger that is rightly to be dreaded.

Pertaining Infrastructure

The function of corporate healthcare infrastructure is usually to provide the platform for effectively utilizing participating systems and devices to support healthcare processes and operations. Therefore, threats and attacks to healthcare Infrastructure target the *Data*, and *Information/Signals* transmitted over them by supported and authorized *Systems* and *Devices*, in order to cripple the organizational *Processes* and *Operations* that rely on them.

These threats and attacks usually adopt methods aimed at reconnaissance and enumeration, intercepting digital/electronic communications, and disrupting services. These methods include wardriving, DoS, APTs, and MITM. In many cases, by the time healthcare Infrastructure comes under threat by malicious actors, the Data and Information transmitted across these Infrastructure are already at risk. This also includes the Systems and Devices that process, store, and transmit these data and information, as well as the organizational Processes/Operations that rely on these activities. Indeed, at this point, there is already a possibility of compromise to one or more of these.

Wardriving is simply the act of searching for Wi-Fi network connections around healthcare facilities from a moving vehicle, and usually with malicious intention. Sometimes, this vehicle could be a motor bike, or a bicycle, in which case, it has often been termed as warbiking and warcycling, respectively. Through this method, malicious actors have been able to discover and latch on to open access connections that integrate private internal networks. Thereby availing a means of dropping malware, spoofing identities on organizational networks, or executing smash & grab operations, in order to steal sensitive healthcare data and information that could be useful for various malicious purposes.

In addition, there is the possibility of applying an MITM technique to effectively search, intercept, and in some cases, tamper with or re-route digital electronic communication. A vast array of tools and techniques have been discovered to feature in MITM operations, including bit-flipping, network sniffers & analysers, and hidden tunnels in network protocols and services. Furthermore, signal jammers/interference generators have also been used to block signals and information that security and alarm systems and infrastructure transmit from sensors/detectors to actuators/effectors.

DoS is a threat-attack approach that works to deny legitimate usage and access to services and utilities (healthcare systems, servers, websites, etc.) either momentarily or indeterminately. One way of achieving this is by keeping these services and utilities engaged in useless and unproductive activities, like processing and responding to packets and requests that amount to nothing. There denying legitimate user requests access to such services and utilities. However, DoS could also be the result of actions and activities by other kinds of malware like ransomware and worms, as well as inadvertent human actions like accidentally disabling connections, or tripping over network hardware. The general idea being that services and utilities are simply unavailable for the purposes of legitimate usage.

Usually, attackers actively seek ways to scale and amplify the impact of DoS operations, and several options are often considered. One of these is to hijack/compromise other user machines within the same infrastructure and bring them under a central-controlled framework by infecting them with a control malware known as a *bot*; and then enlisting them altogether for this malicious operation in a network of bot-infected machines known as *botnets*. Another consideration is to steal the digital identities of user machines within the targeted infrastructure, and then assign these identities to external machines under the attacker's control, before coordinating them altogether for this malicious activity. When a DoS attack enlists distributed support in this way, technically, a Distributed Denial of Service (DDoS) has occurred.

Advanced Persistent Threats (APTs) apply a sophisticated range of stealthy unobtrusive techniques to cover their tracks and evade detection over a prolonged period, after gaining unauthorized access to healthcare Infrastructure. The robust, high-capacity nature of coordination and resources that have been repeatedly discovered to feature in APTs have informed the logical deduction that the threat agents/actors that apply APTs as a strategy are often nation-state entities, or malicious groups that are sponsored by non-state entities. They could target healthcare institutions as a leeway for espionage against larger entities of interest.

The level of coordination that has been seen to feature in APTs reflect their ability to robustly incorporate a vast array of strategies, tools, and techniques across multiple stages that gradually, but systematically build up towards the attack goal or outcome.

Pertaining Processes/Operations

In the context of healthcare, threats to Processes/Operations aim to disorganize and disconcert the security *Resilience*, as well as exploit the security negligence of organizational processes and operations that support *Efficiency*. A common way of pursing this aim is by subversion/bypass of security protocols and routines, usually through naive insider or malicious outsider actions.

Indeed, within the healthcare sector, the design and establishment of processes and operations often aim to preserve efficiency in the organizational business model, as well as imbue resilience against shocks and disruptions. However, in applying these processes and operations towards strengthening and preserving the security status of the healthcare organization, any attempts at subverting or bypassing them have always proven inimical to the long-term security goals of the organization.

Pertaining Policy

Within the cybersecurity threat landscape to eHealth, Policies are rarely the ultimate target of malicious threat actors. However, these threat actors continue to explore the extent of *Robustness* and *Effectiveness* with which policy is able to safeguard organizational assets, processes/operations, and interests, in a bid to uncover exploitable gaps and insufficiencies that offer a malicious advantage.

Often times, attackers pursue this aim through physical events and activities on site at the healthcare facility, and could involve insider operations that are either naive or maliciously intended. Nonetheless, through a systematic process of subverting or bypassing the specifications of policy provisions of healthcare organizations, these threats have often successfully eroded the boundaries and limits of organizational policies, gradually and systematically. In the long run, this exposes and perpetuates critical gaps that could open up paths of little resistance or almost no hindrance at all for malicious actors.

On January 16, 2009, the U.S. Department of Health & Human Services (HHS) and CVS Pharmacy, Inc. – the largest pharmacy chain in the Country – reached a settlement agreement to the tune of $2.25 Million. According to an investigative report, "CVS failed to implement adequate policies and procedures to reasonably and appropriately safeguard protected health information during the disposal process". Further adding that "CVS failed to adequately train employees on how to dispose of such information properly", and "did not maintain and implement a sanctions policy for members of its workforce who failed to comply with its disposal policies and procedures"[7].

The investigation originated following discoveries that CVS casually disposed of pill bottles that contained protected health information of patients (names, addresses, and medication and other personally identifiable information) into open dumps that were accessible to the public. Thereby, potentially violating the privacy of its millions of patients.

This incident provides an insight into the cybersecurity threat landscape that applies to the processes and operations of healthcare organizations, as well as healthcare organizational policies.

What Are the Risk Factors?

There are several risk factors that sometime help to soften the terrain for cybercriminals who target people/users, systems & devices, infrastructure, security lapses in processes and operations, and gaps in policy as a link to lay hands on a healthcare organization's assets. Although, when threats target processes/operations and policy specifications, especially with malicious intention, it is usually as a precursor to a larger scheme, for which success relies on a weakened security culture at the target healthcare facility.

Some healthcare organizations consider basic cybersecurity training as necessary for only their technical personnel or support staff, often citing constraints in funding, as well as the nature of certain job roles perceived to be non-technical. Worse still, many healthcare organizations (particularly across developing countries) fail to employ or regularly contract cybersecurity experts and professionals, even though they feature an extensive repertoire of eHealth products and services. However, when it comes to the context of eHealth, and perhaps other domains of cybersecurity, the role of the keeper and greeter at the entrance to the healthcare facility is as crucial to the protection of cybersecurity as that of the IT manager many floors above.

A doorkeeper that understands how malicious actors might seek unauthorized physical access to healthcare facilities through approaches like piggybacking and tailgating, knows what to watch for when granting access to strangers who fail to promptly and correctly identify themselves at any and all points of entry or encounter within and around the facility. It becomes even better when such an individual also understands the possible resulting risks of implanting hardware keyloggers or network sniffers around the corporate environment.

Similarly, consider a janitor who understands how scavenging for disposed storage devices, sticky notes with personal information, unshredded company documents, or casually disposed corporate systems that are no longer in use could provide malicious actors with useful information to compromise the cybersecurity status of a healthcare organization. Such an individual would be wary of unidentified strangers at intermediate dumpsites or garbage collection points that are used by the organization.

A growing practice that has continued to see people/users, use the same credentials (usernames and passwords) across multiple web services and applications is another potent risk factor that cannot be overlooked. One security report[8] discovered that over 50% of users apply the same credentials across many different web/Internet platforms and services, with another remarkable percentage of these having reused previous passwords over again. The import of this reality for a successful identity theft operation, especially at scale, is indeed non-trivial. For instance, in the event that such credentials of medical professionals who provide services across multiple healthcare organizations are stolen or compromised, attackers could easily leverage these credentials to automate login operations across several popular online healthcare services to breach data and steal electronic patients' health records – in an attack operation known as Credential Stuffing (Figure 2.4).

However, another factor that is a common strain in the subversion of security processes and operations in healthcare, are laxities occasioned by familiarity, naiveness, and nepotism. According to the 20th-Century American Author, Bill Vaughan, "Familiarity is the most destructive of all iconoclasts"; with Professional Coach, Brittany Burgunder, adding that "Just because something is familiar, doesn't mean it's safe. And just because something feels safe, doesn't mean

Target Entity	Threat Objectives	Methods / Approaches / Strategies	Tools / Techniques	Risk Factors
People / Users	Identity theft / digital impersonation; Credential stuffing	Social engineering; Shadowing digital activities	Phishing / vishing; Piggybacking / tailgating; Shoulder-surfing; Keyloggers	Lack of training / awareness; Absence of, or ineffective information verification channels; Using same user credentials across multiple services
Systems & Devices	Reconnaissance / enumeration; Identity theft / digital impersonation; Induced systems / device malfunction; Access denial; Altering data & information	Spoofing; Injection / poisoning; Privilege escalation; Transloading; Drive-by download; Scavenging; Hijacking; Bit-flipping	Malware; Data recovery software; Scanners & trackers; Packet tracers; Cross site scripting (XSS); SQL injection; Bots	Poorly-developed & insecure hardware and software; poor / lack of security culture; More user privileges, access, and accessibility than is necessary
Infrastructure	Digital / electronic interceptions; Reconnaissance / enumeration; Service disruptions	Wardriving; Man-in-the-middle (MITM); Denial of Service; Advanced Persistence (or, APTs)	Network sniffers & analyzers; Hidden tunnels in network protocols & services; Botnets; Smash & grab; Signal jammers / interference generators	Legacy Systems; BYOD arrangements; Offsite / Remote access
Processes & Operations	Erode security culture / protocols / operations	Physical events and activities onsite; Subversion / bypass of protocols and routines		Laxities caused by familiarity, naiveness, & nepotism
Policy				Unawareness & non-enforcement; Absence of robust policies; Poorly-developed policies; Rapid organizational changes; Policy somersault

Figure 2.4   Cybersecurity Incidents in Healthcare – Risk Factors.

it's good for you". Security personnel at a healthcare facility are more likely to subvert/bypass security protocols, processes, and operations, to grant access to an unidentified stranger who has simply become a familiar face at the facility, or to a relative who has not been able to provide authorization to access the facility. In the same way, an employee/user is more likely to be lax about the security of their personal access credentials, data, devices, when a relative or some other familiar person is involved.

Also, a poorly engineered healthcare application that failed to robustly incorporate security protocols and safeguards in its design – like passwords encryption, input validation/error checking, secure socket communication, two-factor authentication, access/logon time-out, etc. – becomes a danger to user data that is collected, generated, or accessed by such an application. Using very simple and unsophisticated tools and techniques, many of them being software that are either freely available on the Internet or have publicly available source codes which only need to be compiled and run, sensitive user data could be siphoned by a malicious external actor.

Then, there are healthcare systems (hardware and software) and devices that do not adopt best practices for security design and hygiene – such as up-to-date anti-malware applications, firewall policies, blockers for ads and trackers, operations that are hardened against interception, as well as interfaces that are resilient to reconstruction – which could become threats in themselves to healthcare data and information. Consider, for example, a security pin pad that incorporates distinguishable key tones, or engineered using hardware that is not resilient against wear occasioned by frequent and repetitive patterns of touch. Over time, this could pose a formidable threat to users' data, access credentials, and other critical information.

In the same vein, there are healthcare organizational policies that fail to guard against, or inadvertently grant to users more privilege, access, or accessibility to organizational systems/devices and infrastructure than is needed to effectively meet the responsibilities of their job roles. This poses an insidious danger to data and information, as these users become direct channels that malicious actors would be more willing to explore in order to reach assets.

In addition, there are the legacy healthcare systems for which manufacturers have published announcements about discovered vulnerabilities; but then, these systems yet unpatched with security releases that fix these vulnerabilities, even while they are still in active use in various healthcare processes and operations. Indeed, this is analogous to a house that is widely known to be without a lock, but is still in use as a store for valuables belonging to various users.

Furthermore, the growing popularity of Bring Your Own Device (BYOD) arrangements means that it is often difficult to achieve a balanced or levelled security status for cybersecurity frameworks implemented in healthcare, since the security of personal user devices cannot be guaranteed off site. Even for organizations with strict policies allowing only corporate devices to participate in their digital spaces, the trend of growing comfortability that frequently sees employees/users treat and handle company devices as their "own property" is a risk that can easily be exploited. Also, off-site/remote-working arrangements often demand that aspects of the healthcare organization's data and infrastructure are accessible off site, such that, at scale, it becomes more difficult to effectively monitor who accesses what, when, from where, and how. All of these realities coalesce to complicate the risk terrain for cybersecurity in healthcare.

The absence of open channels for information verification could also pose a risk factor that enhances the chances of success for malicious actors. In the event of an ongoing attack targeting users/clients and visitors to a newly hosted web-based healthcare service, or a social engineering attempt to steal access credentials for a newly deployed application software, or a rogue/fake business transaction that has spooked a third-party vendor/affiliate. The ability to verify information in real-time through open, and perhaps public-facing channels could spell the difference between success and failure for such malicious incidents.

Again, a culture of people/users' unawareness, non-enforcement of policy provisions, policy somersault, and policy changes that are too rapid and too frequent – these situations have continually posed critical risks to the effectiveness and robustness of policy provisions in safeguarding against the modern realities of the healthcare cybersecurity threat landscape. Policy development processes for healthcare organizations should, of necessity, involve the contributions of cybersecurity professionals for risk assessment. Through new organizational regimes that attempt to bring change too quickly, and especially before the risks and lapses that are ordinarily created by a transitional vacuum are gauged properly, the cybersecurity standing of a healthcare organization can be left vulnerable. Malicious individuals often watch out for these periods of change/transition, as an advantage for orchestrating malicious agenda.

Beyond all these, however, there are also natural occurrences that could equally pose risks to eHealth deployments in healthcare. These occurrences, even though they are often able to bring about the same threat outcomes, differ from the traditional operational regimen of other known Threat Agents. For instance, earthquakes and fires could threaten the operations of backbone technology infrastructure that eHealth applications rely on, such as national telecommunications networks and power grids. While these incidents may pose critical threats to the operations of certain deployments of eHealth – such as unavailability of Internet and telecommunications services for TeleHealth and mHealth applications – they do not reflect the perspective of intent and intentionality that characterizes the operations and activities of traditional threat actors.

Indeed, it can be inundating to come to terms with the true extent and realities of the cybersecurity threat landscape to eHealth and healthcare, generally, especially since what has been discussed and explained in this chapter does not claim to be exhaustive. It is therefore valid to ask, "How can healthcare stakeholders and professionals be better positioned and prepared to cope and engage effectively with these realities?" However, already being aware of the nature and realities of this threat landscape is, perhaps, the necessary first and important step to progress in seeking an answer to this crucial question.

Notes

1 Vectra AI (2020). *The 2020 Spotlight Report on Healthcare*. Industry Research Report. https://content.vectra.ai/rs/748-MCE-447/images/IndustryResearch_2020_Spotlight_Report_on_Healthcare.pdf

2 Check Point (2020). *Cyber Attack Trends: 2020 Mid-Year Report*. https://www.antivirus.cz/Blog/Documents/Check-Point-Cyber-Attack-Trends-2020-Mid-Year-Report.pdf

3 Panda Security (2020, August 26). 43 COVID-19 Cybersecurity Statistics. *Panda Media Centre*. https://www.pandasecurity.com/mediacenter/news/covid-cybersecurity-statistics/

4 World Health Organization (2020, April 23). *WHO reports fivefold increase in cyber attacks, urges vigilance.* https://www.who.int/news-room/detail/23-04-2020-who-reports-fivefold-increase-in-cyber-attacks-urges-vigilance

5 Verizon (2020). *Data Breach Investigations Report (DBIR).* https://enterprise.verizon.com/resources/executivebriefs/2020-dbir-executive-brief.pdf

6 Field, M. (2018, July 20). Cyber-attack on Singapore health database steals details of 1.5m including prime minister. *The Telegraph.* https://www.telegraph.co.uk/news/2018/07/20/cyber-attack-singapore-health-database-steals-details-15m-including/

7 U.S. Department of Health & Human Services (2017, June 07). Resolution Agreement: CVS Pays $2.25 Million & Toughens Disposal Practices to Settle HIPAA Privacy Case. https://www.hhs.gov/hipaa/for-professionals/compliance-enforcement/examples/cvs/index.html

8 Truta, F. (2018, May 03). *59% of people use the same password everywhere, poll finds.* Bit Defender. https://hotforsecurity.bitdefender.com/blog/59-of-people-use-the-same-password-everywhere-poll-finds-19851.html

3

PERSONAL CYBERSECURITY FOR eHEALTH DEPLOYMENTS

Introduction

Adeola is a practising neuro-psychiatric physician at a healthcare facility in Canada. She uses *Psyche-I-Track* – a mobile mHealth application – to track and document the mental health progress of her outpatients. These patients are also able to connect to a patient section of the mobile application to report the status of their mental health at certain scheduled times of the day, primarily by completing an electronic form/questionnaire. They could alternatively have a caregiver or relative do this for them at the scheduled time, when a video-based assessment is not required.

On a workday like any other, for some inexplicable reason, Adeola was suddenly unable to log onto the physician's dashboard of *Psyche-I-Track*. With every attempt to log onto the application, she receives what was apparently an automated firewall response in her official email address. It was a notification communicating her having been shut out of the system, and presented with the option of changing her user password in order to regain access.

Adeola quickly changed her password and logged onto the system in time to meet the scheduled evaluation of her next patient. However, the new password was not very different from the previous one. Actually, both passwords only differed by the addition of a single character in the new password, which was not difficult to anticipate.

Exactly nine days later, a team of experts from Canada's Data Privacy Regulator visit the healthcare facility where Adeola works at, to investigate "suspicious activity" involving patients' electronic health records. At first, the discovery of the incident emerged following anomalous behaviours detected on the Facility's networks from eight days before – since the day after Adeola experienced difficulty logging onto her physician's dashboard on the mHealth application.

DOI: 10.1201/9781003254416-3

The incident had compromised the healthcare data of 11,000 of Adeola's patients; 4,000 out of these had had their electronic health records significantly altered across three different healthcare services provided by *Psyche-I-Track*. Investigations revealed that Adeola's current access credentials had activated the point of compromise that gave malicious external actors an access to the Facility's Infrastructure.

This hypothetical incident provides a pinhole perspective into what has remained the modern struggle of cybersecurity in eHealth – the persistent disconnect between the ability of technology to safeguard itself (effectively and efficiently), and the capacity of human elements to cooperate fully with the security and safety operations of healthcare information and communication technologies. This being a manifestation of the fact that security, with its associated protocols and routines, hardly coalesces well with usability and user convenience. Ultimately, this perpetuates a nagging fear of "who's next, and what's next?" amongst stakeholders in the global healthcare sector – a cloud of uncertainties that has continually shrouded the full potentials of the sector. Which way then? How do we find the balance?

Personal Cybersecurity for eHealth Deployments

Several independent reports (including a 2019 Data Breach Investigations Report [DBIR] by American telecommunications giant, Verizon[1]) have proven that up to 80% of the cybersecurity incidents that occur annually in the healthcare sector, and indeed other domains of information technology application, are directly or indirectly traceable to human lapses in personal cybersecurity.

A range of factors and lapses in personal cybersecurity have been identified as having aided this reality of rife healthcare cybersecurity incidents, including

1. stolen access credentials;
2. weak or unchanged default passwords;
3. tampering with firewall & anti-malware configuration;
4. sharing user credentials (usernames and passwords);
5. altering automatic device and system update settings;
6. uploading wrong or infected files;
7. accessing websites that are unauthorized, insecure, or unsafe;
8. bypassing firewall restrictions for various personal, but naive reasons;

9. transmitting sensitive information over insecure/unverified channels;
10. installing untrusted third-party applications;
11. misusing access privileges;
12. misplaced or shared access to personal/corporate devices and systems;
13. mis-delivering sensitive information to unintended recipients;
14. abuse of access privileges;
15. failing to apply/install updates and patches;
16. clicking links in spam email;
17. failing to promptly identify, and report/escalate threat situations;
18. inappropriately disposing of files and media containing sensitive information;
19. misplaced storage media; and
20. general unawareness regarding best practices for personal cybersecurity, to mention a few.

These are insidious conditions that have proven the bane of personal cybersecurity in the context of healthcare information and communication technologies, the vast majority of which have users/people at the centre of operations.

When you add to these the fact that people/users are often the most vulnerable, most targeted, and most negligent in the high-value eHealth cybersecurity chain, then it probably becomes easier to understand why personal cybersecurity is a non-negotiable for eHealth deployments.

How then can personal cybersecurity be conceptualized and practised in a way that is robust, resilient, and able to meet the contemporary demands and realities of cybersecurity in healthcare?

The answer lies in an understanding of what I would refer to as *"the Intuition for Security"*.

The Intuition for Security

Three characteristics help to describe and define the Intuition for Security. They are *Instinct*, *Knowledge*, and *Behaviour*.

Instinct is the characteristic of rational disposition that catalyses (sometimes subconsciously) a responsiveness to security conditions based on promptings that may be either notional, actual, or experiential.

Knowledge pertains to the capacity for cognizance and discernment, possibly acquired through repeated engagement/association, training/practice, and/or experience.

Behaviour is the characteristic of manifested action(s) that is/are reflective of optimal choice, even in the face of several and usually varied alternative courses of action, which are relatively suboptimal (at least when considered from a security perspective) (Figure 3.1).

These three characteristics help to conceptualize the foundations of personal cybersecurity, especially because, in the practice of personal cybersecurity, Knowledge sharpens Instinct, and both coalesce to guide and inform security Behaviour.

In a most basic sense, it is Instinct that would make a healthcare professional refuse to hand over a work mobile device to a stranger who seems stranded and needs to make an urgent contact. Instead, such individual would rather direct the stranger to a nearby public pay phone service that could be used for the same purpose; or hand the individual some change to use the public pay phone (where financial capability is a consideration); or outrightly refuse to offer any assistance. Even though as an alternative, they could also have handed over a personal mobile device to the stranger for the same purpose, instead.

However, this instinctive behavioural response probably originated from a knowledge of the fact that by dialling a simple USSD code or sending a command by SMS, a spyware or some other malware could be remotely transloaded onto the device. It is also possible

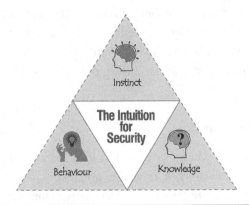

Figure 3.1   The Intuition for Security.

to compromise some other aspects of the device's security status this way. Other events that have been part of the training or experience of the healthcare professional could also catalyse such instinctive behaviour.

Similarly, it is also Instinct that would make a security guard at the entrance to the headquarters building of a large (probably multinational) healthcare organization to ask aside someone who identifies as an employee, but then is unable to gain access to the building because their access card is being rejected by the security system. While putting a call through to the security support unit to request that a staff member of the unit comes to evaluate the situation at the entrance. Whereas, he is also able to manually override the security system and grant access to the individual by bypassing the regular security validation protocol, before directing them to the security support unit several floors above, to lodge a complaint.

However, it is possible that this instinctive behavioural response is catalysed by a previous experience at a regional branch of the organization that saw a stranger gain access to the building without passing the security validation protocol. Before going on to break into the server room two floors above; and, upon detection, was already in the process of copying data from the corporate servers.

In the same way, it is Instinct that would make a medical professional outrightly refuse to lend a removable storage device used to transfer sensitive patient records between hospital systems, to a close friend or relative who needs to transfer data for printout outside the facility. Instead, would rather hand over a personal removable device that does not connect to hospital systems, even though the medical professional could have chosen to move out all sensitive patient data from the work removable device, and then scan the device for malware upon return.

Whereas, this instinctive response might be based on a knowledge of the fact that the work removable device could be recovered of its sensitive data using simple data recovery software tools. There is also the possibility of lacing the device with a novel malware that might go undetected by an anti-malware scan, or swapping (either intentionally, or accidentally) for an identical replica embedded with autorun rootkits.

Therefore, it becomes possible to assess the Intuition for Security, through randomized tests structured to systematically simulate actual threat situations, and then analysing the behavioural choices and responses of the targeted individuals under these test conditions. This would provide useful insights for evaluating the security status of a healthcare organization from the perspective of people/users.

The ability to effectively identify, avoid, isolate, and contain threat agents and threat situations – that is the basic quality of the *Intuition for Security*.

Threat Situations: Identification, Isolation, and Containment

Chapter Two has dealt quite extensively with the various threat agents that could feature in the context of eHealth and healthcare, the operational mechanisms that they have been known to apply, as well as the various threat-attack situations that could be manifested when eHealth deployments are targeted at various levels.

However, the bigger challenge to personal cybersecurity in the context of healthcare and eHealth is how to identify and isolate them, so as to contain their operations effectively, at least at the personal level (where they are wont to target at first), before escalating and reporting accordingly. Indeed, within the context of information and communication technologies, it is virtually impossible to avoid or prevent cybersecurity threat situations entirely. Nevertheless, whether or not they would successfully result in an actual security violation depends, and largely, on being able to effectively identify, isolate, and contain threats and threat agents to cybersecurity from the personal (user-facing) levels of healthcare information technologies.

An understanding of these six principles/guidelines would prove useful, without regard for any particular order (Figure 3.2)

1. Know what assets, over which one has personal or shared responsibility for securing/safeguarding, are likely to be targets and exploited by threat actors. What are the (potential) implications of success for such exploit attempts? That is, what is the security capital of such assets?

   The duties and responsibilities of healthcare stakeholders often necessitate that they assume security custody and stewardship over devices & systems, authentication & access credentials, and physical access control to private workspaces.

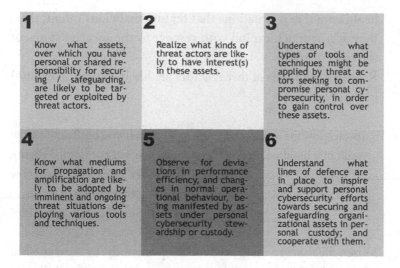

1 Know what assets, over which you have personal or shared responsibility for securing / safeguarding, are likely to be targeted or exploited by threat actors.

2 Realize what kinds of threat actors are likely to have interest(s) in these assets.

3 Understand what types of tools and techniques might be applied by threat actors seeking to compromise personal cybersecurity, in order to gain control over these assets.

4 Know what mediums for propagation and amplification are likely to be adopted by imminent and ongoing threat situations deploying various tools and techniques.

5 Observe for deviations in performance efficiency, and changes in normal operational behaviour, being manifested by assets under personal cybersecurity stewardship or custody.

6 Understand what lines of defence are in place to inspire and support personal cybersecurity efforts towards securing and safeguarding organizational assets in personal custody; and cooperate with them.

Figure 3.2   Six Principles/Guidelines for Personal Cybersecurity in eHealth.

All of which are useful for the various functions of their job roles. In reality, this custody and stewardship extend beyond the physical confines and dimensions of the healthcare organization and facility where these stakeholders operate.

It is imperative to the Intuition for Security that these healthcare players understand the various exploit possibilities against these assets over which they have custody and stewardship. They must also be aware of what success in these exploit attempts could portend for the security status of the healthcare organization – in terms of the security capital that accrues to these various assets with respect to the security status of the organization.

For instance, these could include user credentials for authentication and access, which hold administrative or similar-level privileges; and medical devices that store and transmit contact or healthcare information about patients/clients. It could also include removable drives used for transferring data and information, personal systems and devices that feature in organizational operations as part of existing Bring Your Own Device (BYOD) arrangements, as well as corporate systems that collect, process, and store data about business operations. These assets are among the prime targets in healthcare threat situations that feature malicious intent; thus, they accrue much capital with respect to the security status of the organization.

2. Realize what kinds of threat actors are likely to have interest(s) in these assets.

> If you know the enemy and you know yourself, you need not fear the result of a hundred battles. If you know yourself but not the enemy, for every victory gained you will also suffer a defeat. If you know neither the enemy nor yourself, you will succumb in every battle.
> – Sun Tzu, "*The Art of War*"

When healthcare stakeholders keep custody or stewardship of organizational assets, it is crucial to the responsibility of personal cybersecurity that they are cognizant of not just the value of the assets entrusted to them, but also the kinds of entities that might be interested in laying hold on such assets, especially with malicious intentions.

This is a critical principle for effective personal cybersecurity. One that keeps before healthcare stakeholders the realities about the nature of actors that they are likely to be going up against, as well as what security resources and capabilities are available to defend against these actors effectively. This way, they are better able to gauge and calibrate their Intuition for Security to align with the status and realities of the threat domain they might be entering into by being responsible for securing these assets at the personal level.

For example, a healthcare professional employed at a facility domiciled inside a military or government agency must be cognizant of the fact that even sovereign-affiliated or sovereign-sponsored threat actors might seek to lay a hold on their access credentials and tokens. This could either be useful for accessing secure locations, or secure healthcare systems that might be housing electronic health records of senior government or military officials.

3. Understand what types of tools and techniques threat actors might apply in seeking to compromise personal cybersecurity, in order to gain control over assets. Threat actors usually

deploy a wide range of tools and techniques when they seek to compromise personal cybersecurity as a pathway to valuable assets.

The type of tool or technique deployed usually aligns with the goal or objective that the threat actor seeks to achieve on the journey to the desired outcome. After knowing what assets of personal cybersecurity stewardship are likely targets for threat actors, the next step is being able to understand the tools and techniques that threat approaches and strategies aiming for these assets might incorporate.

For instance, a user being able to understand that a social engineering strategy might incorporate a phishing or vishing technique in an attempt to con users into divulging personal access credentials, or sensitive corporate information, has an Intuition for Security that makes her better able to discern imminent vishing threat situations.

Similarly, a healthcare professional who understands that shoulder surfing is a social engineering technique that might be applied to deduce non-public URLs, and memorize login passwords, and usernames, is mindful about entering personal credentials and accessing private work interfaces on shared computers in crowded public spaces.

4. Know the likely mediums for propagation and amplification for imminent and ongoing threat situations, deploying various tools and techniques. Threat situations, particularly when they have become successful or begun to have a foothold, often explore avenues for propagation, in order to amplify the impact of their malicious operations. Being able to effectively circumvent and immobilize them at this point is perhaps the holy grail of containment goals.

However, as a user, it is not possible to achieve this promptly and effectively without a shrewd (and sometimes in-depth) knowledge of the kind of threat actor involved, and the type of tools or techniques deployed as part of the threat operations. By knowing what type of tools or techniques are being deployed, as well as the methods of propagation or amplification that have been known to be explored by such tools and techniques in operation, it becomes possible to foretell the potential impact of such a threat situation. This makes it possible to forestall or truncate impact effectively, before irreversible or critical damage occurs.

For instance, worms typically propagate autonomously by spreading across devices connected to a network. Thus, an effective approach to circumventing and containing an identified worm threat on a medical system/device connected to a corporate production network would probably begin with taking that device off the network. In the same way, following the detection of a bot infection on a user computer, an effective approach to circumventing the threat operation would probably begin with shutting down remote communications to and from the machine, in order to liberate such a machine from the coordinated control of the remote attacker. These are frequently used approaches, and work reliably. It even featured in a recent report about a June 2020 cyber-attack against Life Healthcare Group[2] – one of the big healthcare organizations in Africa, which operates several facilities across South Africa and Botswana.

However, and particularly as a (non-technical) user, it is important to understand at this point, the far-reaching consequences of such actions. It is also critical to consider the extent possible risk to which certain other organizational processes and operations (some of which could even be security-related) that could result from an action of personal cybersecurity undertaken to safeguard a system or device under threat.

Investigations by the United States Department of Health and Human Services (HHS) Office for Civil Rights (OCR) into a 2010 data breach involving the New York-Presbyterian Hospital (NYPH), was traced to a Columbia University (CU) professor-physician having disconnected a personal device that had been connected to the NYPH network[3]. Apparently, a bilateral relationship between NYPH and CU allowed faculty members of the University to serve as attendant physicians at NYPH, allowing both organizations to co-utilize a data network and firewall service that interfaced with a database server where ePHI (electronically protected health information) was stored.

The professor-physician, who recently developed software solutions for the hospital, had deactivated the device – a personally owned server. However, the absence of effective technical safeguards and organization-wide apparatuses for information risk management consequently resulted in a leak that made some 6,800 patient health information (including vitals, medications, lab results, and overall health status) accessible over the open Internet. In 2014, both organizations had to pay an aggregate of 4.8 million dollars in damage settlement under the Health Insurance Portability and Accountability Act (HIPAA), as an outcome of this non-malicious human action.

Now, there is no evidence to suggest that the action of the professor-physician was a form of threat response, or that the action had a malicious intention, even though investigations revealed that neither of the corporate entities involved had taken adequate steps to ensure that the server was secure and that it contained appropriate software protections. However, this incident does provide insight into the fact that non-malicious and well-intended user actions, even when geared towards enhancing safety and security, could ultimately prove inimical to corporate security interests, especially without having considered such actions robustly and shrewdly.

So, ultimately, if any user actions at circumventing threat situations would be considered effective in the long run, then the appropriate technical support and security teams of the healthcare organization must be promptly and expeditiously notified at the point where such actions are being considered in the very first place, or immediately such actions are executed (in the worst case). This would help avert disruptions in downstream business operations that might be reliant on the disabled workstation, and which could be equally critical to business processes and the security status of the organization.

5. Observe for signs of deviation in performance efficiency, and changes in normal operational behaviour by assets under personal stewardship or custody. Diminishing performance efficiency or sudden changes in normal operational behaviour are common obvious manifestations of impending and ongoing threat situations – often characterized by noticeable

deviations in the normal patterns of efficiency, performance, and operational behaviour.

For instance, when systems and devices suddenly begin to slow down with ads and prompts sprawling about, or network connections and services begin to throttle or fail, or the abrupt lockout of authentication and access credentials. If there is no other higher-level technical explanation for these occurrences, then they could well be indicative of ongoing malware exfiltration or MITM operations on packets, data, and information. They could also signal malicious attempts to compromise the availability of network-based services for accessing client data; and efforts aimed at impersonating an authorized digital identity, respectively.

Indeed, a perceptive Intuition for Security would be one that is quick to suspect these occurrences as having possible malicious undertones.

6. Understand what lines of defence are in place to inspire and support personal cybersecurity efforts towards securing and safeguarding organizational assets in personal custody, and cooperate with them. These lines of defence could exist in settings on systems, software, and devices; infrastructure configurations; policy provisions; or established security protocols/processes/operations.

For instance, some healthcare organizations configure robust device policies on corporate systems and devices, some of which enable remote tracking and/or erasure of certain classes of devices that fail to connect to the secure corporate infrastructure every few hours. Others have in place, robust firewalls and systems for intrusion detection and prevention, as well as routines for automatic backups on a periodic basis. There are also those that maintain up-to-date corporate-level anti-malware products and services. In addition, there are equally healthcare organizations that deploy very strong password and authentication policies (including two-factor authentication, and logon timeout) across the board, or across certain critical levels of user operations. Likewise, there are healthcare organizations with device sign-in policies that photograph users and automatically activate device tracking after a maximum number of failed sign-in attempts.

All of these are some lines of defence that might be in place to help inspire and support personal cybersecurity efforts in the context of eHealth, either by way of complement, or supplement for security resilience and threat prevention. Hence, it is important that healthcare professionals are familiar with, and cooperate with these lines of defence as part of the process of enhancing their Intuition for Security in order to engage effectively with the modern realities of the cybersecurity threat landscape for eHealth.

Therefore! Use strong passwords, and change them regularly. Avoid reusing old passwords, regardless of how long it has been since the last usage. Quickly install/apply security updates soon after they are released. Do not share or reveal personal access credentials. Refrain from fiddling with security software and utilities, for which the capacity to operate knowledgeably is lacking. Be wary of clicking links and bypassing filters to visit web locations or download resources that are ordinarily restricted, or possibly flagged as potentially dangerous. Be careful when performing sensitive work functions/duties using personal devices. Do not write passwords and access credentials on pieces of paper; digital password management software offer a safer alternative. These are to mention a few.

Now, there could be dreadful situations when self-preservation is a consideration for personal cybersecurity such as when life and personal safety might be directly under threat. Under such circumstances, understanding what lines of defence are available to support personal cybersecurity could trigger behavioural responses that would, in retrospect, reflect optimal choice for personal cybersecurity, in a way that does not endanger personal safety.

Therefore, towards being able to identify, isolate, and contain threat situations to personal cybersecurity in healthcare applications of information technology, it is not just enough that healthcare stakeholders know what assets under their security stewardship are likely to be exploited by threat actors. They must also be able to realize what threat actors might have interest in gaining a foothold on these assets, and equally understand what types of tools and techniques threat actors are likely to apply in seeking to compromise these assets. Beyond these, however, it is important to observe for deviations in performance efficiency, in order to be able to circumvent threat situations by immobilizing mediums for propagation and amplification. Whereas, all of these rely on a shrewd understanding of what lines of defence are in place to support and inspire personal cybersecurity efforts.

Escalation and Reporting

It is a fact that there are certain threats and threat situations to personal cybersecurity in the context of healthcare information technologies, for which ordinary (technically untrained) stakeholders might be unprepared or unable to deal with effectively. Consider, for example, those threat situations that involve sovereign-sponsored or sovereign-affiliated threat agents and entities, or even actual sovereign entities themselves. Where threat resource capabilities abound and often far exceed the best of whatever might be in place to support and inspire personal cybersecurity.

In such situations, it is foolhardy for users to assume that they might be able to engage effectively and resiliently with these threat situations. Hence, part of the responsibility of personal cybersecurity in eHealth, and indeed the Intuition for Security, is being able to identify when one is up against a threat actor that, by far, out-matches their resource capabilities (e.g. training, and security setup), and knowing when and how to escalate and report appropriately.

Nonetheless, it is indeed crucial to escalate that all suspected, confirmed, successful, or unsuccessful threat attempts against personal cybersecurity. It is important to report such attempts promptly and adequately to the relevant units/mechanisms within the healthcare organization. To disregard this is dangerous, because it is seldom the case that threats to personal cybersecurity are lone or random incidents. They are often coordinated attempts to compromise the cybersecurity status of an organization/enterprise on a large scale. Thus, by reporting such attempts promptly and effectively, it becomes possible to activate adequate measures of vigilance early enough to forestall imminent large-scale attacks.

However, the approach to Incident Reporting and Escalation is fundamentally a function of what organizational or regulatory structures are in place to manage cybersecurity incidents (either as a specific class of incidents or as part of a generic incident-handling repertoire). Therefore, the establishment of structures and mechanisms for effective incident handling and management is non-negotiable for healthcare organizations, especially considering the critical nature of operations that characterize healthcare services delivery, and the dimensions of risk to human life. Beyond this, it is equally important that People/Users are aware of procedures specified by organizational incident management mechanisms for incident escalation and reporting.

Nonetheless, the struggle to communicate cybersecurity incidents effectively to the appropriate organizational technical support, and security or incident management teams is one that is real for both the non-technical users (who often report these incidents) and the technical teams who have to respond to these incidents. This is many times the result of a disconnection between how well users are able to communicate the incidents in the escalation reports, and how understandable and useful these reports are to inform timely and effective technical responses. Here are a few illustrative questions to help People/Users effectively escalate and report healthcare cybersecurity incidents to technical support and response teams.

a) How would you describe the realities of your personal cybersecurity and user experience in the recent period preceding the onset of the incident up until the time of reporting?

Be sure to state all occurrences of note that you might have experienced as an information technology user in the period leading up to the time of reporting the incident.

These might be notable happenings or occurrences in personal engagements, involvements, and interactions for which there was an (attempted) interface with devices, systems, or access credentials.

b) Are there any noticeable changes or deviations in normal operating behaviours and conditions of information technology assets under personal custody? Have these events ever occurred before?

Ensure that all noticed abnormalities relating to the personal use of information technologies are adequately stated.

Do not forget to state having previously noticed these abnormalities, if that is the case.

c) What user operations and activities were in progress before the onset of these behaviours?

Report aptly the operations and activities pertaining to the personal use of information technology that were ongoing about the time the first and subsequent abnormalities in behaviour and operating conditions were noticed.

d) Were there any surrounding circumstances of note that were associated with the incident?

If there were any associated events, be sure to state these as well. These events could have been environmental, functional/operational, or otherwise.

e) Were any personal (authorized or unauthorized) measures taken prior to the time of escalation/reporting, concerning the situation(s) being escalated/reported?

Be sure to state precisely and transparently what personal measures might have been taken previously with regards to the incident being reported, regardless of whether such measures were authorized or not. Also, mention what insights might have informed these measures.

f) Were there any previous attempts to escalate/report such events and occurrences?

In case previous attempts have been made at escalating or reporting such events and abnormalities, either formally (through existing organizational channels) or informally, be sure to mention such as well, also ensuring to state what were the outcomes or directives that emanated from such attempts, if any.

g) Do you have any current suspicions and opinions about the incident under reporting? What might have informed these suspicions/opinions?

It is okay to have personal suspicions and opinions regarding the incident under reporting. After all, you were arguably a point of initial contact for that incident. Hence, state these suspicions clearly and unequivocally; and do not forget to mention what might have informed these suspicions.

It is probably a good idea to have ready answers to these questions in oral reports of cybersecurity incidents. Even with written incident reports, it is equally important to ensure to provide answers to these illustrative questions within such written reports. These illustrative questions do not claim to be exhaustive; however, they do provide a useful guide for effective progress in this regard.

It, therefore, becomes evident that personal cybersecurity in the context of healthcare and eHealth is only effective to the extent that organizational mechanisms are in place to:

a) ensure up-to-date training and awareness for users;
b) provide robust security policies and protocols that fortify the security status of the organization;
c) guarantee real-time information verification, as well as technical support that is prompt and efficient;
d) manage and minimize risks and liabilities effectively and circumspectly; and,
e) establish resilient processes and procedures for coordinated incident reporting, escalation, investigation, response/handling, and recovery.

This is further instructive of the fact that the journey to effective personal cybersecurity begins at the higher levels of administration and management of the healthcare organization or institution. Because it is only within this framework that the effects of mindfulness for cybersecurity would be able to ripple across and downwards from the higher levels, in order to strengthen the capabilities for personal cybersecurity by sharpening the Intuition for Security.

In light of the current realities of eHealth cybersecurity, it has long ceased to be a question of "if" a healthcare organization and her assets are going to come under threat at any point, but rather a question of "when", and "how" a healthcare organization and her assets would come under threat. Thus, it boils down to the measures and steps put in place to enhance preparedness and responsiveness in the face of imminent or occurring threats and attacks to an organization's cybersecurity status. How well they would perform under threat situations is a direct function of how security-ready they are at the time the threat manifests.

Notes

1 Verizon (2019). *Data Breach Investigations Report (DBIR)*. https://enterprise.verizon.com/en-gb/resources/reports/dbir/2019/healthcare/
2 Life Healthcare Group (2020, June 09). *The Life Healthcare Group regrets to announce that its southern African operation has been the victim of a targeted criminal attack on its IT systems*. https://www.lifehealthcare.co.za/news-and-info-hub/latest-news/life-healthcare-announces-cyber-incident/
3 McGee, M. K. (2014, May 07). $4.8 Million Settlement for Breach: Heftiest HIPAA Penalty Yet from Federal Regulators. *Data Breach Today*. https://www.databreachtoday.com/48-million-settlement-for-breach-a-6822

4

DATA/INFORMATION
SECURITY FOR eHEALTH
DEPLOYMENTS

Introduction

From the *General Data Protection Regulation* (GDPR) of the European Union, to the *Health Insurance Portability and Accountability Act* (HIPAA) of the United States, the *Protection of Personal Information* (POPI) Act of South Africa, the *Personal Information Protection and Electronic Documents Act* (PIPEDA) of Canada, the *Digital Information Security in Healthcare Act* (DISHA) of India, the *Act on the Protection of Personal Information* (APPI) of Japan, and *Kenya's Health Act*, 2017, all of these Acts and Regulations reflect the great importance that is placed on healthcare data/electronic health records in many jurisdictions around the World.

In 2013, *Advocate Health Care*, an Illinois-based healthcare facility, was constrained to pay civil settlement claims to the tune of $5.55 million, to HHS' Office for Civil Rights for violations of the HIPAA[1]. Through a chain of incidents that began in August 2013, multiple breaches resulted in the electronic patients' healthcare information (ePHI) of 4 million individuals being compromised. Data that were breached included names, demographic information, addresses, credit card numbers, dates of birth, clinical information, and health insurance information of the affected patients.

In one of the incidents leading up to this breach, Advocate Medical Group, a subsidiary of the healthcare organization, had suffered a burglary at one of her offices that resulted in the stealing of four laptop computers containing patients' information. In another incident, an external access to the organization's network compromised the healthcare information of 2000 patients. In yet another incident, a work laptop computer was stolen from the vehicle of an employee of the Organization. All the incidents took place between August and November of 2013.

Whereas, healthcare regulations and acts in many jurisdictions place upon healthcare organizations that collect, process, transmit, and store patients' electronic medical records, the responsibility of ensuring that these data are kept safe, secure, and accessible, even within the ambience of binding regulatory specifications. To falter in this responsibility typically amounts to a regulatory violation that has often been responded to with huge fines and large settlement pay-outs.

Indeed, this responsibility translates to mean that healthcare organizations have a duty to manage data in the most effective and efficient manner that ensures that data elements are (a) trustworthy and reliable for informing medical decisions, (b) kept safeguarded against unauthorized encounters and interferences, in·order that privacy is preserved, and (c) guaranteed to be promptly available at all times, at all such points, and for all such uses, functions, and operations that are authorized, ethical, and lawful.

In Chapter One, the Invariants of Healthcare Data have been presented and discussed. But then, in the practice of modern healthcare, how do these Invariants reflect the premium that is placed on them by various healthcare stakeholders – regulators, patients/clients, healthcare service providers, healthcare professionals, and third-party vendors/affiliates. What approaches can be applied to help minimize risk and liability from a non-technical standpoint, so that healthcare organizations and professionals are better able to navigate the non-trivialities of regulation? This is the grain of discussions in this chapter.

Data/Information Security for eHealth Deployments

Data and Information Security remains critical for eHealth deployments, particularly because the sensitive nature of data that is electronic patients' health records is one which is hedged by a complex strain of considerations pertaining to Human & Digital Rights, Democracy & the Rule of Law, Personal Security, Public Health & Safety, and National Sovereignty.

For instance, the right to personal dignity must be preserved even for individuals who are suffering terminal ailments, and might even be at the point of death. The multi-stakeholder frameworks of regulatory specifications governing how healthcare data are to be handled, accessed, and managed must also be circumspectly adhered to. The handling and management of patients' healthcare data must align with wider acceptable best practices, as well as the best interests of the greater public. The security of persons who are patients and suffering certain medical conditions may also often rely on keeping their healthcare records private and secure. While sometimes, healthcare data and systems could equally provide an avenue through which external interference could threaten the sovereignty of a state.

However, at the centre of this quagmire of complexities is a consensus regarding the fact that electronic health records or patients' healthcare data are to remain reasonably trustworthy, accessible, private, and protected against interference, disclosure, usage, processing, transmission, as well as other data-related operations and interactions that are unauthorized, especially such that fails to directly and transparently secure the informed consent of the data subjects themselves. In several jurisdictions, independent regulatory agencies have been established to safeguard and ensure the Invariants of Healthcare Data, by operating and applying a body of prescriptions and specifications enshrined in Acts, and Regulations.

For healthcare organizations, the struggle is not just with respect to compliance with existing regulations; it also pertains to building a reputation of transparency and fiduciary responsibility in service delivery. The growing awareness of the duty of healthcare organizations to ensure adequate as well as effective security and risk management for electronic medical data and information, coupled with the regulatory roles that have been played in catalysing this awareness, and the responsiveness of government to infractions and violations in many jurisdictions, reveal the non-trivial nature of this struggle.

Even though several governments (such as the United States) have established frameworks for incentivizing "meaning use" of technology in domains such as healthcare, the regulatory repercussions for failing to meet the requirements specified for safe, secure, and responsible applications can quickly dwindle the utility and advantage that such incentives offer.

Integrity, Confidentiality, and Availability: Invariant and Non-Negotiable

Integrity, Confidentiality, and Availability play a crucial role in the utility that eHealth offers for global healthcare. Indeed, their role is indispensable. As highlighted in Chapter One, this can be attributed to a number of factors and realities. Here are a few of them that have played out in happenings within the global healthcare sector in not-too-distant times passed.

In 2017, eClinicalWorks, a cloud-based electronic health records system that provides vendor services to healthcare organizations in the United States from Westborough, Massachusetts, was reported[2] to have been facing a class action lawsuit of close to $1 billion for certain irregularities that were detected in the data operations of the system, which made it difficult for data readings on the system to be trusted – potentially endangering the lives of patients. The lawsuit alleged reliability concerns in the health information of potentially millions of victims, which made it difficult to consider such information as being trustworthy.

These allegations included periodically displaying incorrect medical information charts on patient screens, periodically displaying medical information for multiple patients concurrently on a single view, failing to display medical history accurately on progress notes in specific workflows, as well as audit logs that failed to accurately record user actions, alleging a breach in fiduciary responsibility and gross negligence on the part of the healthcare vendor – eClinicalWorks.

This incident reveals the importance of reliable and trustworthy data and information operations to the business of healthcare delivery. Indeed, whenever the veracity of medical data and information becomes in doubt, then the utility of the eHealth operations and process chain is truncated for the entire case in focus (whether they be products or services). This also portends potentially harmful implications for life and safety. Therefore, it is little wonder that the ECRI Institute (formerly, Emergency Care Research Institute) in a 2019 Report[3] highlights data integrity issues in EHRs among the top concerns for patient safety in healthcare organizations.

A 2018 incident[4] also saw a public hospital in Portugal slapped with a fine of €400,000 by the Comissão Nacional de Protecção de Dados (Portugal's Supervisory Data Protection Commission) for a violation of the European Union's GDPR. In this incident, investigations revealed that a deficiency in the profile management system of an eHealth service resulted in 985 registered profiles of medical doctors, even though the hospital had only 296 doctors.

This meant that a wide range of healthcare workers and professionals – (non-medical) staff, psychologists, dietitians, and other professionals, through false profiles, were able to access the electronic medical records of patients, even for those patients that had nothing to do with their medical speciality, healthcare work, or duty of employment.

In this incident was revealed the non-negotiable fact that healthcare data and information are to be kept only accessible to authorized individuals who need such data to perform certain well-defined healthcare or medical functions that serve the best interests of the data subjects. While also ensuring that informed consent is received with respect to how such data would be accessed and used.

Another case that involved *Cignet*, a medical service operating multiple healthcare facilities in southern Maryland, USA, pertained to 41 patients who had requested access to their healthcare records between September 2008 and October 2009. The healthcare organization had failed to meet this request for several months. Even though specifications in the HIPAA, at the time, required that healthcare institutions provide a patient with a copy of their medical records within 30 days, and no later than 60 days from the time a request is received.

On March 30, 2010, a default judgement was obtained against *Cignet* Health of Prince George's County, Maryland, by the U.S. Department of Health and Human Services' (HHS) Office for Civil Rights (OCR), for violating several regulatory specifications of HIPAA. Even though *Cignet* had managed to produce the medical records to OCR on April 7, 2010, this was several months past the required deadline specified by HIPAA. *Cignet* was slapped with a civil money penalty of $1.3 million for this violation.

While the reason for this default was not clearly established in this case, the incident does provide a clear perspective into the imperative of ensuring that medical records are available at all times when they are requested or needed.

In another incident[5] that was reported as arguably the first actual death that can be directly traced to the impact of a cyber-attack, a patient died at a hospital in the city of Düsseldorf on the night of September 11, 2020. A ransomware attack the previous day had compromised the Hospital's systems by exploiting a vulnerability in the Citrix virtual private network (VPN) system being used at the Hospital. Thus, the hospital was unable to admit the female patient in emergency, who was suffering a life-threatening illness, because they were locked out of their systems and could not access her medical records. The ambulance carrying the patient was diverted to Wuppertal, 30 km (20 miles) away, and she is said to have died on the way there.

Through the eyes of this incident, perhaps, it further becomes clearer why availability is an invariant of healthcare data, and why healthcare regulations place a remarkable premium on the imperative of ensuring rapid access and response in matters pertaining to the availability of data and information in the context of healthcare.

Although not explicitly stated in all cases, these example cases are apparently the result of incidents that can be directly or indirectly traced to design flaws in system and software engineering that perpetuated critical cycles of vulnerabilities, malware actions that may have gone undetected, insider threats for which motive and intention may not have been accurately deduced, or an absence of robust and efficient security safeguards for data and information. Altogether, however, they reveal the necessity of ensuring that in all deployments and applications of eHealth in global healthcare, privacy is safeguarded, integrity is preserved, confidentiality is ensured, and availability is guaranteed. How then can these be pursued in the light of current realities?

Preserving Integrity

It is no gainsaying that the essence of information technology (or eHealth) applications in healthcare has been primarily for the purpose of ensuring that access to quality healthcare services is available ubiquitously and without any form of confinement or incapacity that is imposed as a result of geographic location, mobility, or similar constraints. Whereas, the utility that is provided in this context relies on medical/healthcare data and information being available in just the same manner, and particularly in a way that can be trusted as accurate and reliable for informing medical/healthcare diagnosis and decisions.

All of these crumble when Integrity is compromised. So, how then can Integrity be ensured in healthcare applications of information technology (eHealth)?

1. One school of thought that has been widely considered in this regard is allowing patients (frequent/periodic) access to their healthcare/medical data. The reality of device sensors with wide error margins, as well as the possibility of interceptions and alterations that could occur at different points in the data processing/operations chain are facts that have been more evident by recent events. By allowing patients access to their data at various points in the processing/operations chain, it adds a layer of interest-based verification that can be relied upon as the chain continues to scale. The logic is pretty simple: no one can be more interested in the accuracy of medical/healthcare records than the patients themselves.

   However, this does not in any way diminish the responsibilities attributed to healthcare organizations for safely collecting these data and information, as well as processing and storing them in a reliably secure manner. Therefore, in no respect can this layer of verification be construed to mean a shift or relegation of this responsibility.

   It is also important to realize that hackers can be patients too (or pose as one). Hence, security measures must be in place in this context to verify the identities of individuals (patients) requesting access to healthcare data over eHealth deployments, and also to ensure that these individuals (patients) are only able to access their data, their data alone, and nothing but their data.

   Biometric authentication has frequently been explored as a foolproof way of verifying individual identities for this purpose. Additional measures like firewall restrictions, honeypots, and intrusion detection/prevention systems, have also been applied in several contexts to restrict what can be accessed and viewed under such circumstances, while also watching for anomalous behaviours that are suggestive of malicious intent and operations.

2. Maintain log files at various points in the data processing and operations chain, for the purpose of tracking and checking whenever errors are suspected or confirmed. Audit logs are indispensable to the goal of ensuring integrity in the management of electronic medical/healthcare data and information. This is because in many cases, when infractions are being investigated, audit logs provide a way of establishing or disproving corporate irresponsibility on the part of the healthcare organization. Beyond this, it also helps healthcare organizations during routine checks, to be able to flag red points in their operations and process chains, which could compromise their risk standing.

All of these are possible because audit logs help to trace the points of origin when integrity issues emerge. It provides a means of identifying what might have been the cause of such issues, as well as determining what technical, structural, or operational measures would have helped avert such occurrences at the organization-wide level.

Safeguarding Privacy

Even though the term "privacy" continues to feature in discussions around healthcare cybersecurity incidents, the term itself has no universally accepted definition, except such as is defined within the context of regulations that are binding in particular jurisdictions. This is because privacy, in its essence, has more personalistic dimensions with overlapping considerations that regulations often struggle to capture adequately in a single body of specifications. These include bodily integrity, personal dignity, secrecy & seclusion (that is, identification, non-identification, or selective identification), and agency/individual autonomy, to mention a few. The major struggle of regulations is to balance the various interests of all privacy stakeholders across these several dimensions.

However, privacy remains a top consideration whenever infractions occur against healthcare/medical data and information. In essence, when healthcare cybersecurity incidents happen, stakeholders seek to establish whether the trust reposed in healthcare organizations to effectively safeguard and secure the patients' data and information that they collect and hold in confidence has in any way been downplayed, so as to ascertain how efficiently they had fared in this responsibility.

Privacy policies help to align the business interests and goals of healthcare organizations with the responsibility of safeguarding privacy. Even though beyond this, healthcare organizations are often additionally required by regulation to have in place a robust risk management plan that would help them to proactively assess, detect, mitigate, and respond effectively to risks that endanger patients' medical data and information.

Furthermore, regulations in certain jurisdictions (such as the GDPR of the European Union) have specified best practices aimed at preserving privacy from an organizational-to-user standpoint. These include

1. Removing personally identifiable information from healthcare/medical data that are collected about patients, and sometimes mapping these to pseudo-identities or special tokens that help to uniquely distinguish records pertaining to particular individuals within digital operations and processes, without necessarily identifying such individuals personally – a technique known as *Anonymization/Pseudonymization*.
2. Collecting very limited amounts of data and information that can be used to uniquely identify patients, which is intuitive because the lesser the amount of personal data and information that is required of patients who patronize healthcare services, the easier it is to keep such personal data and information undisclosed (since disclosure imposes upon the one to whom is being disclosed, the responsibility of preserving privacy), thereby reducing the surface areas of potential internal and external threats – a technique known as *Minimization*.
3. Ensuring that privacy considerations are embedded into the very foundational stages of conceptualizing, designing, and engineering software and systems for use in healthcare – an approach known as *Privacy by Design*.

Privacy by Design can be pursued by making certain that (a) the most stringent privacy settings are activated by default in new systems and software (otherwise called *Privacy by Default*), (b) proactive privacy measures are incorporated, so that risks to privacy can be anticipated and forestalled even before they materialize as breaches/incidents, (c) end-to-end security techniques are applied to enforce privacy throughout the life cycle of data processes and operations, and (d) sensitive data and information are computed and processed securely at all times, at all points, and for all purposes. These are to mention a few.

But then, Privacy and Confidentiality share a rather interesting relationship. While Privacy is the end, Confidentiality is the means. In other words, it is the imperative of safeguarding Privacy that imposes upon healthcare organizations the responsibility of ensuring Confidentiality.

Ensuring Confidentiality

With respect to Confidentiality, healthcare organizations have a duty to protect the electronic healthcare/medical records of patients from unauthorized access, even from within the organization itself. This demands that patients' data and information are only available to those professionals and workers who require access to these records either for effective medical diagnosis or to enhance the quality of healthcare delivery. It also requires that measures are in place to ensure that these healthcare/medical professionals and workers are unable to disclose such data and information without authorization, and consent of the subject.

To compromise confidentiality, even internally, is to dwindle general confidence in the ability of a healthcare organization to effectively safeguard EHRs from threats that could come from any medium, including externally. This has often been the focus of regulatory repercussions that follow when confidentiality is compromised. How then can confidentiality be preserved?

The basic principle for ensuring confidentiality is Access Control. However, how this is applied could sometimes vary according to the state of the data/information being safeguarded (whether it be at rest, or in transmission). Nonetheless, the conceptualization of approaches is broadly the same, since the goal is generally to ensure that unauthorized entities are unable to access, extract, or view data and information that is considered confidential.

1. Access Authentication to Confirm Authorization of Requesting Entities.

   In trying to safeguard confidentiality for patients' data and information in eHealth, it is important that sensitive medical records are only accessible to those who are authorized. This usually implies adding a layer of authentication, as a process of confirming the authorization of entities requesting to gain access to such data or information.

   Combining this with an event log operation further helps to track and know which entities accessed what particular data or information, and at what time, also making it possible to determine what user operations have been performed on sensitive data and information, even by authorized entities.

2. Encryption to Enable Secure Transmission, Storage, and Retrieval.

   Encryption is basically the process of ensuring that sensitive data and information can ordinarily not be read or interpreted as it is. This is typically achieved by encoding sensitive data and information in a form that requires a secret key or passphrase in order for the data or information to resolve back to a plain readable form.

   When this technique is applied across the entire spectrum of data communication/transmission processes, it is referred to as end-to-end encryption (or, E2EE).

Guaranteeing Availability

In several jurisdictions, regulations often require that patients are provided with access to their healthcare records within a specified maximum time period. This requirement is specified either as part of a healthcare regulatory act, or as part of a general citizens' information/data regulatory act. Within these jurisdictions, the inability to meet this requirement by providing patients with access to their healthcare data within the specified period (and for any reason whatsoever) amounts to a regulatory violation that has often been met with huge fines and settlements.

But then, how can availability be guaranteed in the context of eHealth and healthcare information and communication technologies, generally? A number of methods and approaches that have been widely adopted include creating and managing backups, adding redundancy, as well as carrying out periodic maintenance on systems, devices, and services, in order to tune the performance for data processes and operations.

1. Basically, backing up is a technique that helps to guarantee availability through the replication of data elements, resources, and utilities. Through this technique, sensitive healthcare/medical data and information are replicated to ensure that they remain available even in the face of threats like malware actions, database corruption/malfunction/failure, or loss due to deletion.

2. Redundancy is closely related to the concept of backing up. Except that, while backing up often pertains to data elements, resources, and utilities; redundancy is more relevantly applied to infrastructure, systems, components, and functions. Redundancy refers to the duplication of critical infrastructure, systems, components, and functions in order to enhance reliability by creating a fail-safe alternative that guarantees availability.

   However, a common mistake that is often made in the creation and management of backups and redundancies is that of not taking care to ensure that they are not exposed to the same risk factors as those in use. For example, domiciling a backup media on site at the healthcare facility, and under the same conditions as in-use data media, could expose such backups to the same risk factors like fires, theft, malware attacks, insider threats, etc. The same applies to redundant infrastructure, systems, components, and functions.

   In many cases, cloud-based options have been recommended, as it not only removes the backups and redundancies from the physical/environmental risks that could threaten the utilities that they provide, but it also makes these backups and redundancies available without restrictions to geography or location. But then again, there is also the need to be cognizant of the fact that cloud backups and redundancies do not automatically and entirely transfer the responsibility of data and information security to cloud vendors, although, regulations have sometimes considered a shared and well-defined parity arrangement in this regard.

This is first because cloud infrastructure, platforms, and services are usually provided on an "*as-is*" basis, and subscribing organizations have the responsibility of configuration and customization by adding and dropping features in order to meet their security standards and needs and also because cloud platforms have been discovered to be a new target domain for cybercriminals[6].

3. Tuning operations basically avail a means of optimizing the performance of data sources, and database services, and by extension, the data processes and operations that rely on them, thereby ensuring that they continue to function optimally, effectively, and efficiently. At scale, this becomes particularly important, as the implications of having to wait for indeterminable periods of time as data processes and operations progress through sub-optimal paths could be critical for both healthcare organizations and their patients/clients.

To this end, it is additionally important that periodic maintenance operations are carried out on eHealth systems, devices, and services. Such as disk error checking to fix bad sectors, memory defragmentation to optimize memory operations, reviewing error reports and firewall policy/event logs to spot anomalies and warning signs, inspecting hardware integrity to identify defects and deficiencies that could result in failure, updating security features and applications, applying system upgrades and patches, clearing files that are no longer in use to free up disk space, as well as running scans and diagnostics to detect and analyse system faults.

Other considerations for circumspect data and information security in eHealth are to scrutinize and audit data sources, data elements, and databases that are assimilated through mergers, acquisitions, and business consolidation. Sometimes, these assimilations could bring in vulnerabilities and risks that are able to jeopardize the security standing of the parent organization and pre-existing data assets.

Periodic penetration tests that simulate actual cyber-attack conditions and operations also help to provide useful insights into the security resilience of organizational frameworks, structures, processes, and policies. These are crucial for identifying fault lines that threaten data and information security and could upturn the security status of healthcare organizations that deploy information and communication technologies for healthcare/medical service delivery.

Furthermore, there is also the need to ensure that third-party vendors, subsidiaries, and affiliates are held accountable to the same data and information security standards as that of the parent healthcare organization. Many a time, it has been seen that lapses from these third parties have wittingly or unwittingly created and perpetuated vulnerabilities that ultimately impacted negatively on the parent organizations.

Ultimately, the security of data and information in the context of eHealth remains a responsibility of healthcare organizations, which cannot be abdicated, at least in the sight of regulation. In bringing in various other players and actors to interface with healthcare information and communication technologies, the risk surface is expanded for healthcare organizations, even though the responsibility remains sacrosanct. When these players and actors understand the measures and mechanisms that are applied to ensure integrity, safeguard privacy, preserve confidentiality, and guarantee availability, they are better able to cooperate with, and support existing measures and mechanisms towards desired goals and outcomes.

Notes

1 Becker's Healthcare (n.d.). Advocate to pay largest HIPAA settlement to date. https://www.beckershospitalreview.com/healthcare-information-technology/advocate-to-pay-largest-hipaa-settlement-to-date.html

2 McGee, M. K. (2017, November 20). *$1 billion lawsuit focuses on EHR data integrity concerns: Suit against eclinicalworks alleges millions potentially harmed by use of software.* Information Security Media Group, Corp. https://www.bankinfosecurity.com/1-billion-lawsuit-focuses-on-ehr-data-integrity-concerns-a-10463

3 ECRI Institiute (2019, March 11). *Diagnostic Errors and Test Results Top ECRI Institute's Patient Safety List: New report pinpoints risks from EHRs, mobile health, behavioral health, clinician burnout, and more.* https://www. ecri.org/press/diagnostic-errors-test-results-top-patient-safety-list

4 de Meneses, A. O., & Quathem, K. V. (2018, October 26). Portuguese Hospital receives and contests 400,000 € fine for GDPR infringement. *The National Law Review, VIII*(299). Covington & Burling LLP. https://www. natlawreview.com/article/portuguese-hospital-receives-and-contests-400000-fine-gdpr-infringement

5 Reuters in Düsseldorf (2020, September 18). Prosecutors open homicide case after cyber-attack on German hospital. *The Guardian (United Kingdom).* https://www.theguardian.com/technology/2020/sep/18/prosecutors-open-homicide-case-after-cyber-attack-on-german-hospital

6 Ashford, W. (2018, July 13). Hackers increasingly targeting cloud infra-structure. *Computer Weekly.* https://www.computerweekly.com/news/252444716/Hackers-increasingly-targeting-cloud-infrastructure

5

SECURING eHEALTH SYSTEMS AND INFRASTRUCTURES

Introduction

According to the *Cost of a Data Breach Report 2020*[1] published by IBM, data breaches cost the global healthcare industry alone an average of USD 7.13 million annually, with up to 90% of healthcare organizations that featured in a 2016 survey[2] by Ponemon Institute having experienced a data breach in the preceding two years, and each organization losing an average of USD 3.7 million of revenue per data breach. The reputational impact of a healthcare cybersecurity incident has also been discovered to last for between ten months to two years[3].

So, in considering together the loss of revenue, the loss of customer/client trust, the diminishing of Industry reputation, and the uncompromising strictness of regulation, it quickly becomes obvious how the impact and implications of cybersecurity incidents for healthcare organizations are too non-trivial to hyperbolize. To disregard these critical realities by a healthcare organization could, very well, be likened to an act of self-immolation. But then, what imperatives are necessary for robustly securing eHealth systems and infrastructures in the practice of modern healthcare?

Securing eHealth Systems and Infrastructures

Security has been defined as "the procedural and technical measures required (a) to prevent unauthorized access, modification, use, and dissemination of data stored or processed in a computer system, (b) to prevent any deliberate denial of service, and (c) to protect the system in its entirety from physical harm"[4]. Rightly so because, in practice, security that is robust and effective is one that incorporates measures to ensure

DOI: 10.1201/9781003254416-5

Securing eHealth Systems & Infrastructures			
Physical Imperatives	Logical Imperatives	Operational Imperatives	
♦ Restrict access to offices and workspaces. ♦ Preserve the integrity of the organizational environment. ♦ Adopt avenues and options for secure disposal.	⇒ Limit the coverage and accessibility of eHealth systems & infrastructure. ⇒ Maintain an up-to-date security status for eHealth systems and infrastructures. ⇒ Partition access to eHealth systems, infrastructures, and data resources according to various functions, operations, and use cases. ⇒ Restrict the interactions and participation of personal digital devices with eHealth systems and infrastructures.	♦ Adopt a gradual integrated approach to technology changes and transformations. ♦ Establish policies and processes using bottom-up approaches that are multi-stakeholder-involved. ♦ Build and nurture a strong cybersecurity culture. ♦ Create an internal framework / mechanism for risk assessment and incident management.	Monitoring and Evaluation for Compliance

Figure 5.1 Cybersecurity Imperatives for Securing eHealth Systems and Infrastructures.

the integrity and reliability of data and information, prevent malicious attempts at disrupting services and utilities provided by systems and infrastructures, as well as safeguard the external/environmental setting wherein these systems and infrastructures function.

Intuitively, therefore, Security in the context of eHealth essentially incorporates physical, logical, as well as operational aspects. Each of these aspects has implications for the four dimensions of cybersecurity previously highlighted in Chapter One – Infrastructure & Systems, People/Users, Processes, and Policies. How then can cybersecurity be ensured for eHealth systems and infrastructures, both physically, logically, and operationally, and without disregard to the multi-dimensions of robust cybersecurity? (Figure 5.1)

Cybersecurity for eHealth: Physical Imperatives

A frequent misconception has been to assume/think that cybersecurity has only non-physical aspects and implications. However, several cybersecurity incidents that have been witnessed in the domain of healthcare in recent times have proven that the journey to compromising cybersecurity could well begin from the physical perspective. In the same way, as the path towards a formidable and long-term solution to healthcare cybersecurity incidents has sometimes involved simply fixing a causative or pre-disposing trend/reality in the physical dimension. Here are some physical imperatives that can be reliably applied toward securing eHealth systems and infrastructures.

1. Restrict access to offices and workspaces. It is important that personal workspaces are only accessible to the healthcare and medical professionals who work in these spaces, or other employees of the healthcare organization (in case of shared workspaces). Allowing non-employees access to these workspaces, or even granting unfettered access to other employees who ordinarily do not share these workspaces, poses an insidious cybersecurity threat to healthcare organizations.

   Insiders could have access to data, information, systems, devices, or infrastructural facilities that are above their privilege levels, while outsiders (even without provable malicious intent) might be inadvertently allowed into a space wherein they are unable to adequately fathom the critical high-risk nature of operations and realities. In addition, medical and healthcare professionals should be especially wary of leaving patients alone and unsupervised/unattended during private consultations, or leaving their systems and devices unattended during working hours, because cybercriminals can be patients too.

2. Preserve the integrity of the organizational environment. Loosely hanging network (Ethernet) cables, uncovered or broken pattress boxes and cable trunking, cabling that runs pretty long (sometimes, publicly accessible) distances to connect end-to-end, digital/electronic devices lying around within environs of healthcare facilities, which bear no identity nor can be accounted for – all of these are common environmental sights around many healthcare organizations that have implications for cybersecurity. Hardware packet sniffers, keyloggers, signal jammers/interference generators, and network extenders/repeaters have been able to successfully latch onto eHealth systems and infrastructure through these means, without being detected for considerably long periods of time.

   Therefore, when cabling has to run considerable distances and wireless options are not preferred, conduit channels are a recommended option. But then, when the physical integrity of these channels is compromised, they must be fixed expeditiously. Similarly, network cables that are not/no longer in use should be de-crimped and stopped, or uninstalled altogether.

Furthermore, it is good practice to conspicuously brand digital/electronic devices that are owned and operated by healthcare organizations, particularly ones that function internally (within the organization's facility). This makes it easier to identify alien ware when they are spotted within the healthcare facility.

3. Adopt avenues and options for secure disposal. Indeed, it would not be any gainsaying that much of the electronic waste generated by healthcare organizations potentially contain sensitive data and information that cannot be casually disposed of. This includes storage media, systems, devices, and even non-electronic hardcopy printed documents and inscribed pieces of paper. Hence, it is important to establish adequate measures and procedures to securely dispose of such materials when no longer useful or in use.

    For recyclable and non-recyclable electronic materials, organizational measures should be established to ensure that they are completely ridded of the data and information that they contain (or used to contain), so that they are non-recoverable, or at least not easily recoverable. Similarly, non-electronic materials should be effectively shredded and/or incinerated as well.

Cybersecurity for eHealth: Logical Imperatives

The 2019 Spotlight Report on Healthcare[5] by artificial intelligence industry leader – Vectra AI, Inc. – revealed how the status of certain in-use systems and infrastructures continue to pose insidious cybersecurity threats to the utilities that information and communications technologies bring to healthcare. Echoing well-known challenges with the use of information technologies in critical industries like healthcare, associated with (a) networks and similar infrastructures that are not properly partitioned along various functions, operations, and use cases, (b) access control measures that do not (or no longer) provide adequate and effective security, as well as (c) long delays in rapidly deploying updates and upgrades to existing systems and infrastructures.

The result is a perpetuated threat situation that has many times seen eHealth systems and devices with vulnerabilities that have long been publicized by manufacturers and developers, still featuring actively in healthcare operations, even though measures have not been taken to ensure that they have received the most up-to-date security patches and fixes. Also, there is a potentially dangerous situation wherein a central production network/database infrastructure serves both employees, guests/clients, as well as third-party vendors & subsidiaries of healthcare organizations, without effective boundaries and limits. In addition, there has also been the reality of critical production systems and infrastructures being used in various healthcare functions and operations, reaching far too widely without adequate safeguards against external interference.

Therefore, as part of the logical imperatives for effectively securing eHealth systems and infrastructures, it is important to

1. Limit the coverage and accessibility of eHealth systems & infrastructure. It has often proven inimical to the interest and goals of cybersecurity of information technology in healthcare for organizational systems and infrastructure to be accessible beyond the scope wherein coverage is required for authorized use. Broad-range wireless networks that are still accessible hundreds of metres away from the healthcare facility, files and folders shared on healthcare systems to be accessible over poorly secure networks, remote connection capabilities that are not end-to-end resilient against interception and tampering, including eHealth systems and devices that are able to pick up insecure (and unverifiable) wireless network signals from several metres outside the healthcare facility – these are common logical vulnerabilities that have plagued eHealth systems and infrastructure in the modern digital era.

   As a basic principle, it would be neither an exaggeration nor paranoia to recommend that all (sensitive) data and information that feature in the context of eHealth and healthcare information technologies generally, are encrypted and only transmitted over secure communication channels. Indeed, this is already required by a number of jurisdictional regulations for healthcare data and personal information generally, some even explicitly.

Beyond this, digital coverage and accessibility of eHealth systems and infrastructure should be checked and controlled effectively. As a rule, it is important to ensure that such systems and infrastructure that routinely handle data and information which could be both sensitive and critical, are not accessible beyond the scope of reach wherein they are required for authorized functions and operations.

2. Maintain an up-to-date security status for eHealth systems, infrastructures, and data resources. Adequate organizational measures should be put in place to ensure that an up-to-date security status is maintained for eHealth systems and infrastructures at all times through periodic upgrades and updates within timeframes that are reasonably short enough to reflect an effective security posture against the existing threat landscape. The Australian Cyber Security Centre (ACSC)[6] recommends a maximum duration that ranges from 48 hours to 30 days after a patch is released for it to be applied to vulnerable systems and information technology assets, depending on the specified risk level of the associated vulnerability – 48 hours for extreme risk, 14 days for high risk, and 30 days for moderate-to-low risk.

Furthermore, it is important that the eHealth systems and devices that are used to process, store, access, and transmit sensitive patient healthcare information feature resident shields and firewalls that prevent them from connecting to or transmitting over open access/public/unverified network connections. Email servers should also be configured with built-in security software that checks email attachments and links to verify their safety. These are imperative for creating layers of logical barriers that are necessary to protect sensitive healthcare data and information from malicious external actors seeking outbound (exfiltration) or inbound (infiltration) access to such data and information by breaching eHealth systems and infrastructures.

Supported by a generous adoption and systematic deployment of other cybersecurity hardware and software utilities, such as end-point anti-malware solutions, intrusion detection and prevention solutions on systems and networks, digital alarm/tripwire systems, etc., a formidable security status can gradually be pursued for eHealth systems and infrastructures.

3. Partition access to eHealth systems, infrastructures, and data resources according to various functions, operations, and use cases. Visitors and clients at healthcare organizations should not ordinarily be able to access the same network connections as medical professionals and workers at the facility, neither should third-party vendors. Subsets of central systems and infrastructures should be created to serve various compartmentalized functions, operations, and categories of users. For instance, virtual private networks (VPNs) used for internal communications should be kept encrypted, reserved for this purpose, and only accessible to authorized entities. When aspects of healthcare operations are outsourced, it also becomes necessary to segregate the nature, extent, and involvements of such relationships.

The database systems and infrastructure that store sensitive patient healthcare data and information should also not be directly accessible to certain classes of users, especially those that are non-technical. Intermediate pre-processing mechanisms have often been used in reviewing requests for access/connection, and deciding whether these requests could otherwise be serviced by a subset of the central database system/infrastructure. This helps to preserve efficiency, and also forestall a situation wherein a bad user command or request might endanger a database asset of the organization.

Furthermore, access to eHealth systems and infrastructures, as well as the data that they handle, should be oriented towards the tasks and job functions of various roles. Front desk workers do not need access to patient health records beyond that which pertains to scheduling their appointments. In the same way as Pharmacists might not necessarily need access to patient medical/healthcare records beyond that which relates to their medication history.

4. Restrict the interactions and participation of personal digital devices with eHealth systems and infrastructures. Bring Your

Own Device (BYOD) arrangements have sometimes offered a leeway through which threats and attacks have compromised the security of eHealth systems and infrastructures. The extent to which the security status of personal devices that interact with eHealth systems and infrastructures can be ascertained, is often limited to the extent to which organizational policies can effectively regulate the operations and activities of such devices across other engagements and interactions. In many cases, it is difficult to achieve such effectiveness in a foolproof way.

Medical doctors who prefer the convenience of using their personal mobile devices to access eHealth portals and interfaces for prescribing patient medications, patients who use personal computers for TeleHealth consultations with healthcare professionals, and off-duty medical practitioners who use personal computers to pull medical records of monitored patient cases – all of these interactions and participation of personal digital devices in eHealth, are latent threats to the security of information technology systems and infrastructures in healthcare.

It is therefore important that healthcare organizations that operate such BYOD arrangements have well-defined logical rules and policies that clearly specify and restrict what kinds of operations, interactions, and functions are authorized for such devices that feature within their healthcare services and operations chain, especially when patients' sensitive healthcare or medical information is involved.

Cybersecurity for eHealth: Operational Imperatives

Healthcare organizations that feature eHealth systems and infrastructures in their chain of services and operations shoulder a huge responsibility. It is that of ensuring that the practices, procedures, and activities that characterize their organizational approach to operations and services do not become inimical to the interests and goals for cybersecurity of the eHealth systems and infrastructures that they rely on. How can healthcare organizations ensure that the cultures and regimens that characterize their services and operations do not threaten the cybersecurity status of eHealth systems and infrastructures? Here are a few suggestions of operational imperatives to help safeguard the interests and goals of healthcare organizations in this regard.

1. Adopt a gradual integrated approach to technology changes and transformations. Periods of change and transformation are often characterized by vacuums that can be occasioned by (a) insufficiencies/deficiencies in the scope of knowledge and information across several ranks, (b) uncertainties regarding what the future is likely to bring about (c) the struggles to adapt to disruptions to the *status quo*, and sometimes the inadequacies of existing coping mechanisms, and (d) (perceived/actual) insufficiencies in current individual or collective capacities and capabilities to meet the demands of the new era. These are some of the socio-technical realities that have frequently been associated with technology-related changes and transformations.

   Hackers and cybercriminals watch out for such periods of changes and transformation too, and are quick to spot lapses that could be exploited to compromise security. One testament is the sudden transition to working from home for many organizations as a result of widespread lockdowns across the World occasioned by the COVID-19 Pandemic of the year 2020[7]. The rapid digital transitions exposed many healthcare organizations to threats and attacks from cybercriminals, who, evidently, were already lying in wait.

   Thus, it is important that changes and transformations, especially those that are technology-related, adopt a gradual integrated approach – one that is coordinated and keeps in focus, the fundamental socio-technical realities of the organization, beginning from the baselines. Through this approach, users can be inspired and supported to gradually grow into technological changes and transformations, in ways that would be beneficial to the goal of holistic outcomes that impact positively on business interests.

2. Establish policies and processes using bottom-up approaches that are multi-stakeholder-involved. A key lesson that has

been learnt in the course of civil class actions and huge settlement fines over the course of recent years is that the responsibility of ensuring cybersecurity for eHealth systems and infrastructures is not reserved exclusively for the Chief Security Officer (CSO), the Chief Information Security Officer (CISO), or the Security & Risk Management Apparatuses of the healthcare organization.

One of the most embarrassing realities that have been experienced by several organizations in the discourse of healthcare cybersecurity, and indeed cybersecurity generally, is how the huge investments that have been applied, and shrewd strategies adopted at the higher levels of the organization to formulate policies and processes that are both robust and resilient, all fall flat at the baselines of the organization with the naive click of a button.

In essence, it is never bad counsel to involve the lower ranks of the healthcare organization in discussions pertaining to the establishment of new policies and processes, and the revising of old ones. This is imperative since human errors and mistakes resulting from unawareness regarding cybersecurity best practices adopted by healthcare organizations – which are often enshrined in corporate documents that define organizational policies, processes, and procedures – is one of the leading socio-technical and socio-cultural lapses that have continued to plunge the global healthcare sector into unnecessary cybersecurity distress. In fact, it was the leading causative factor behind 90% of cyber data breaches that were reported in the United Kingdom in 2019.

3. Build and nurture a strong cybersecurity culture. The cybersecurity status of an organization is only as resilient as the overall cybersecurity culture that is reflected at all levels of the organization. In the healthcare industry, and actually all industries, a robust cybersecurity culture can often spell the difference between an averted threat situation, and a successful cyber-attack. But then, how can such a culture be built?

Inspiring a robust approach to vigilance that is inclusive, and incorporates a zero-trust (that is, trust none and verify all) model is, perhaps, a good way to start. Ultimately, all stakeholders of the healthcare organization must become partners and collaborators in the responsibility of corporate cybersecurity, supporting and complementing each other through the sometimes inconvenient best practices and approaches to securing healthcare information and communication technologies. Reward and compliment good security behaviours and practices, by tracking even those that are not physically manifested, and also ensure to promptly correct and remedy bad security behaviours and practices, in the same way. Establish cybersecurity policies (e.g., password and user account policies, firewall and remote communication policies, device control policies, etc.) and ensure to enforce them.

Beyond these, however, and perhaps more importantly, an atmosphere must be created wherein users and employees feel comfortable reporting unwitting actions or lapses that might have inadvertently compromised the security status of the organization, or violated certain security policies, even when such security compromises are merely notional, and may not yet have resulted in an actual security incident. Within such an atmosphere, healthcare organizations might be able to buy useful time to respond or react effectively, which could help them avert greater consequences from imminent security incidents. However, without an atmosphere wherein people/users feel comfortable revealing such lapses without fear of undue reprimand, such gains would be difficult to achieve.

But then, in order for any of these to be as effective, training, awareness, and capacity development must cease to belong in the exclusive domain of the technically competent individuals for whose job functions and roles these might be required. Rather, let every stakeholder be reasonably aware of what the cybersecurity apparatus of the organization looks like, what safeguards/restrictions are in place, and where; what measures for monitoring and accountability have been established; what are the levels of tolerance for security risks; what information technology assets are critical for defending, and the nature of threats to be defended against; which entities and domains are high-risk; what to do when under threat or attack. It is important that no stakeholder is left behind in any of these regards.

Now, it might be argued that this basically hands the pie to a malicious insider. However, when considered holistically with the body of other physical, logical, and operational imperatives, it becomes obvious that a cybersecurity culture is but a complementary aspect, which is as crucial as every other in the task of safeguarding eHealth systems and infrastructures.

4. Create an internal framework/mechanism for risk assessment and incident management. This is indispensable for the business of healthcare service delivery because risks and incidents to eHealth systems and infrastructures could directly portend grave implications for the safety of life. Thus, healthcare organizations need to have in place a framework/mechanism for internally assessing cybersecurity risks and managing incidents before they wreak undesirable outcomes on the organization.

   This would particularly help healthcare organizations to gauge effectively the implications of certain processes, operations, and practices for long-term business continuity, while also enhancing and strengthening their capacity to detect, investigate, prevent, respond, contain, and recover from cybersecurity incidents with minimal damage and losses.

   But, even more importantly, these frameworks/mechanisms should be robust, proactive, and responsive enough to spot cybersecurity risks before they actually become incidents. Possibility, likelihood, consequential impact/severity, mitigability (by degree), and avoidability. These are well-known pillars of effective risk assessment – being able to establish the possibility that an incident could occur in context, the likelihood that it would occur (given the existing organizational processes, operations, and practices), the impact/severity of the resulting consequence, how such impacts could be diminished/diffused, and to what degree, and the extent to which such a risk can be avoided altogether. These are critical considerations for the cybersecurity of eHealth systems and infrastructures.

Furthermore, a resilient operational contingency plan is indispensable to the risk management and incident response apparatus of healthcare organizations that deploy eHealth systems and infrastructure. This would be helpful in ensuring that healthcare operations are not ground to a halt when risks transform into incidents.

Monitoring and Evaluation for Compliance

Unfortunately, none of these physical, logical, or operational imperatives would be as effective without a coordinated approach to monitoring and evaluation, in order to ensure compliance at all levels of the healthcare organizations where eHealth systems and infrastructures feature in various capacities. A monitoring and evaluation plan has often proven useful in helping to structure and guide efforts and activities in this regard.

This usually begins by defining what are the goals/outcomes of monitoring and evaluation efforts, how these goals/outcomes are to be benchmarked, as well as what compliance entails (with respect to indicators, and how they might be measured/assessed in context). Perhaps, and for example, measuring compliance could be envisaged in terms of successful regulatory (re-)assessments, or in terms of a decrease in the number of passwords flagged by account management systems and servers as not compliant with the organization's password policy requirements.

All of these can then be formalized into a plan that outlines what approaches and methodologies would be deployed towards the monitoring and evaluation process – which could be physical, logical, or operational – and how these would be applied. Next would be to decide what evidence(s) would be pursued, based on the benchmarked goals of the monitoring and evaluation plan, before employing the necessary resources that are needed to ensure a smooth and efficient monitoring and evaluation process.

Indeed, it is the approach to monitoring and evaluation for compliance that creates the ambience of proactiveness and responsiveness, which, in the long run, enhances the capacity of the healthcare organization for effective security of eHealth systems and infrastructures.

However, in order to proceed knowledgeably in this regard, an intuitive first step is being able to understand what digital ecosystems exist around new and current deployments of eHealth, and how these ecosystems function and interface with the digital capacity and assets of the healthcare organization.

Understanding Ecosystems of eHealth Deployments

As was highlighted in Chapter Two, when eHealth deployments begin to scale and expand, it is often seen that new digital ecosystems of healthcare operations and services begin to form around existing frameworks and processes. Understanding the implications of these new ecosystems for existing structures, particularly with regards to data and information security, is critical to the success of healthcare organizations in these ventures.

What new ecosystem(s) of digital interactions are created (or expanded) by this new scope of healthcare service or operation? What elements participate in this new ecosystem(s)? What dimensions of cybersecurity need to be taken into consideration, in order to effectively safeguard operations within this new healthcare digital ecosystem(s)? These are fundamental questions that are critical to understanding the ecosystems that form around eHealth systems and infrastructures.

A client base in a new jurisdiction, a new branch or subsidiary, a new vendor/supplier/affiliate, a new healthcare service, a new employee, transitions in working arrangements – all of these are activities that healthcare organizations could undertake, which open up new ecosystems around existing eHealth deployments.

Within these new ecosystems, it is important to be cognizant of new data access points that are created, extensions of existing digital infrastructures (networks & systems), acquired/integrated digital participants and assets (data, systems, users), as well as new regulatory implications that might have been imposed by these new ecosystems. All of these new realities must be properly enumerated, and should form part of the considerations for monitoring & evaluation plans and efforts, especially in order not to perpetuate redundant ecosystems around eHealth systems and infrastructures that could surreptitiously avail an entry point of least resistance to malicious actors.

Therefore, access credentials that are created when employees are hired, must be deactivated and archived when an employee ceases to work at a healthcare organization anymore. When users switch between eHealth services, their access to previous services should be disabled. Network and data access points for former vendors and affiliates should be promptly shut down. When working-from-home arrangements change, the remote provisioning and access to certain eHealth resources and utilities should be reviewed accordingly. Digital devices and storage media belonging to the healthcare organization should be retrieved when medical professionals change employers.

Taken holistically, these few pointers highlighted in this chapter offer a progressive template that could be robustly applied towards better cybersecurity for eHealth systems and infrastructures in the practice of modern healthcare.

Notes

1 IBM (2020, July 29). IBM Report: Compromised Employee Accounts Led to Most Expensive Data Breaches Over Past Year. *IBM News Room*. https://newsroom.ibm.com/2020-07-29-IBM-Report-Compromised-Employee-Accounts-Led-to-Most-Expensive-Data-Breaches-Over-Past-Year   (c.f. https://www.ibm.com/security/digital-assets/cost-data-breach-report/#/).

2 Ponemon Institute (2016, May). *Sixth Annual Benchmark Study on Privacy & Security of Healthcare Data*. Research Report. https://www.ponemon.org/local/upload/file/Sixth%20Annual%20Patient%20Privacy%20%26%20Data%20Security%20Report%20FINAL%206.pdf

3 Experian (2012, January 27). *Ponemon Institute Study: Reputation Impact of a Data Breach*. https://www.databreachtoday.com/whitepapers/ponemon-institute-study-reputation-impact-data-breach-w-540

4 Turn, R., & Ware, W. H. (1976). Privacy and security issues in information systems. *The RAND Paper Series*. Santa Monica, CA: The RAND Corporation. https://www.rand.org/pubs/papers/P5684.html

5 Vectra AI (2019, April 24). Report: A vulnerable attack surface exists in healthcare enterprise IT networks. News Release. https://www.vectra.ai/news/2019-healthcare-spotlight-report

6 Australian Cyber Security Centre (ACSC) (2012, April 01). *Assessing Security Vulnerabilities and Applying Patches*. https://www.cyber.gov.au/acsc/view-all-content/publications/assessing-security-vulnerabilities-and-applying-patches

7 European Union Agency for Network and Information Security (ENISA) (2020, May 11). *Cybersecurity in the healthcare sector during COVID-19 pandemic*. https://www.enisa.europa.eu/news/enisa-news/cybersecurity-in-the-healthcare-sector-during-covid-19-pandemic

GOVERNANCE, ETHICS, AND REGULATION IN EHEALTH

Introduction

The imperatives of governance, the responsibilities of ethics, and the oversight of regulation: These are three characteristics that make the adoption of eHealth for modern healthcare particularly challenging for many jurisdictions, especially the fact that governance structures (both at the national and international levels) should be robust and inclusive enough to engender wider unanimity with regards to the duties and responsibilities of healthcare organizations that deploy information and communication technologies, while also ensuring that broad-based compliance is achieved with regards to all the multi-stakeholder regulatory specifications and requirements that apply to the deployment of eHealth for modern healthcare. Oftentimes, the difficulty for healthcare organizations also arises as a result of trying to balance corporate/business interests against the ethical duty of pre-serving trust, transparency, and accountability in the various applica-tions of eHealth, and under the oversight function of regulation.

Nonetheless, and in the light of the current realities that continue to transpire in this space, the distinguishing factor for success or fail-ure of healthcare organizations that adopt healthcare information and communication technologies, relies to a great extent on the effective-ness of the internal frameworks of such organizations in (1) align-ing corporate interests with the broader consensus of governance as pertains to eHealth, (2) minding that the operations of healthcare information technologies agree with the wider-acceptable duties and responsibilities of ethical practice, and (3) ensuring compliance with all binding regulations that pertain to the adoption and deployment of eHealth.

The goal is to ensure an effective balance between (a) the structures and functions of administrative frameworks for internally governing

DOI: 10.1201/9781003254416-6

the operations of eHealth in alignment with business interests, (b) the wider-acceptable ethical duties and responsibilities of adopting healthcare information technologies, and (c) the unavoidable necessity of compliance with multi-stakeholder regulatory requirements in this regard.

For healthcare organizations, the persistent reality of threats lingering ever so near, in a very dynamic and unpredictable threat landscape, imposes an added layer of wariness that becomes rather too risky to relegate, ultimately resulting in a convolution of imperatives that must be robustly considered in seeking to deploy eHealth in ways that would not ultimately prove inimical to business sustainability and continuity in the long term.

However, the journey to achieving this effective balance and blend of governance, ethics, and regulatory compliance in the applications of information and communications technologies to healthcare begins by understanding the various goals and considerations that apply to governance, ethics, and regulation in the context of eHealth.

Governance, Ethics, and Regulation in eHealth

Governance, in the context of eHealth, refers to the various structures, functions, and patterns of authority, engagement, and multi-stakeholder involvement that are applied towards safeguarding the utilities of healthcare information and communication technologies. According to the World Health Organization (WHO)[1], Governance with respect to eHealth entails certain duties and responsibilities across national and global levels.

At the national levels, Governance is said to involve directing and coordinating the development and applications of eHealth, building consensus and multi-stakeholder equilibrium around policy, and protecting individuals and groups by providing an assurance of oversight and accountability in the various applications of eHealth. Whereas, at the international/global levels, it pertains to discourses around the rights, responsibilities, rules, and risks that apply to various stakeholders in the use of global technology utilities (such as the Internet) for purposes that relate to healthcare, the handling and management of sensitive healthcare data, and the application of other information technologies for healthcare.

In its most excellent form, approaches to Governance should be "participatory, transparent, accountable, effective and equitable", through the application of processes that promote the rule of law. But then, the governance of eHealth continues to face several challenges on the path to making this a reality: one being the well-known difficulty of achieving consensus and equilibrium on various issues amongst stakeholders with interests that are often both competing and conflicting. Also, and often as a fallout of the preceding point, there is the challenge of trying to sustain momentum for progress and action when change is supposed to be multi-stakeholder driven.

The implications of governance at the organizational level for healthcare institutions remain equally non-trivial. However, despite the proven cost-effectiveness of using information technologies in healthcare, and the accompanying benefits of efficiency, scalability, and portability, several healthcare institutions continue to struggle to consistently reap these benefits because internal governance structures, functions, and operations are often fractured at the centre. Indeed, it is fairly easy to boil down cybersecurity incidents in healthcare information technologies to lapses and insufficiencies in structures and frameworks for governance at the organizational level.

For example, incidents that are traced to user unawareness or inadvertencies can be directly or indirectly linked to lapses in organizational structures for building knowledge and capacity, managing risks, or responding to threat situations. A similar attribution can be applied when vulnerabilities in systems and infrastructures result in cybersecurity incidents.

The nature of discussions around **Ethics** in the context of eHealth, does not particularly differ from that which pertains to the operations and services of healthcare delivery in general. It refers to the imperative of ensuring that the applications of eHealth do not trample the wider-acceptable standards, norms, and values that characterize appropriate behaviour, actions, choices, and decisions. Discussions around Ethics in eHealth could exist across two broad panels/schools of thought: prescriptive (that is, as defined by standardized bodies of laws, norms, and social customs) and normative (that is, based upon certain fundamental rights, obligations, and responsibilities that are inalienable and exist at the very essence of humanity).

In its most excellent form, ethical considerations in the applications of healthcare information and communications technologies continue to explore an effective blend of the prescriptive and normative schools of thought in a progressive and consistent manner. However, a frequent challenge often emerges when prescriptive considerations begin to exclude and obscure the normative realities of Ethics. This is a concern that has continued to malign the proven utilities of eHealth in many jurisdictions.

However, there exist certain well-established and widely accepted principles that have been discovered to be indispensable to the ethical applications of eHealth. They include:

a) Autonomy: the ability to think, will, choose, decide, and act independently, without any form of external inducement or coercion.

    Thus, eHealth should not interfere in any way with the capacity of subjects (patients or other human agents) to decide/reverse after deciding, to choose/refuse to choose, or to act/refrain from taking action.

b) Privacy & Confidentiality: the right to seclusion that takes into consideration the choice to be identified, selectively identified, or unidentified (that is, privacy), and the responsibility of ensuring the preservation of this right (that is, confidentiality) in all patient-related healthcare interactions.

    Thus, in the applications of eHealth, the healthcare subjects must be able to evaluate and authorize what is/would be known about them, at every point in time.

c) Human Dignity: the realization that certain unique values and attributes that are intrinsic and inalienable to the essence of the human person, bestow a worthiness of respect on such a person that is not dependent on any other factor(s).

    Thus, in delivering healthcare services through eHealth, it is non-negotiable that respect for the person who is the patient is upheld at every point.

d) Informed Consent: the obligation of ensuring that subjects are enabled to make decisions on a voluntary and knowledgeable basis, empowered by an in-depth understanding of what might be the (several) outcomes and implications of such decisions.

At all points of the interface where information and communication technologies would be applied for healthcare service delivery, patients should be made aware of what would be the nature and implications of their involvements with eHealth, what risks are involved, as well as what measures have been taken to mitigate such risks, in order that their decision to get involved with eHealth is well-informed.

e) Justice and Fairness: the moral obligation of ensuring that actions, processes, and outcomes are honourable, and adjudication is based on equitable considerations, even when interests and claims are competing/conflicting.

This requires that when disputes and conflicts arise in healthcare applications of information technologies, equity should be preserved through unbiased adjudication.

f) Beneficence & Non-maleficence: the mindfulness of being cautious that the welfare of the subject is preserved at all times and at all points where eHealth is applied for healthcare service delivery, by avoiding to do harm either by way of intention, negligence, or inadvertence.

This necessitates that eHealth is deployed such that it does not in any way harm the patients either directly or indirectly.

However, Ethics, as it pertains to eHealth is known to face a number of challenges. One such challenge relates to ethical definitions that are sometimes essentially too ambiguous to apply across several different contexts and use cases without conflict and confusions around notion and intent. Then there is also the challenge of circumstances that are superimposed by existing realities within the scope of eHealth applications in particular jurisdictions – such as the digital divide and technology capacity maturity, which could entrench and exacerbate perceptions of inequalities in medical and healthcare services that are provisioned through eHealth. These are to mention a few.

Regulation in the context of eHealth deployments is the application of the force of legislation in establishing and demanding compliance with certain critical requirements that are necessary for safeguarding the development and utility of various applications of eHealth in the delivery of healthcare services within and across particular jurisdictions.

Its utility exists in being able to provide the level of assurance that engenders the wider adoption of eHealth within and across jurisdictions, by preserving trust, transparency, and accountability for all stakeholders in the healthcare services chain. The stakeholders in this regard being (a) patients (who could be citizens or non-citizens), (b) healthcare professionals who provide medical and non-medical services, (c) regulators, funders/investors, and administrators, (d) insurers and vendors.

Thus, discussions around the Regulation of eHealth centre on (1) the safeguarding of personal healthcare and medical information from such collection, storage, or processing that is not/no longer consented to – that is, *Data Sovereignty & Privacy*, (2) protecting sensitive healthcare data and medical information from unauthorized disclosure/exposure, alteration/corruption, and unavailability/loss – that is, *Data Protection*, (3) preventing unfair and indignifying practices against stakeholders in the provisioning, sales, processes, and operations of eHealth products and services by justly specifying liabilities, rights, and responsibilities – that is, *Consumer Protection* (or *Provider/Manufacturer Liability*), and (4) enforcing standards to spotlight and prevent anti-competitive conducts and operations amongst stakeholders in eHealth services – that is, *Fair Competition*.

But then, what are the fundamental goals that drive and sustain the utility of regulation in the context of eHealth? An understanding of these goals, and the challenges that are frequently encountered in the pursuit of these goals, is crucial to fathoming the responsibilities of management and administration that are attributable to healthcare organizations with regards to eHealth.

Understanding the Goals and Challenges of Regulation

One factor that presents a fundamental consideration for the regulation of eHealth is the fact that eHealth challenges and trumps traditional models of healthcare service delivery whereas, traditional healthcare service delivery is characterized by physical presence at points of service that are predetermined, with a progression through the system of service delivery that is quite direct and well-defined. eHealth adopts a more dynamic and unconstrained path for various modes/levels of healthcare service delivery (primary, secondary, tertiary, and quaternary), which is not otherwise limited by physical boundaries.

Within this context, the goal of regulation is to clarify the nature, establish the extent, and safeguard the integrity of interactions that take place wherever eHealth is applied in the delivery of healthcare services. Such interactions could be (a) between patients seeking healthcare/medical services and the practitioners who render such services, (b) amongst healthcare practitioners in the duty of rendering healthcare/medical services, (c) between healthcare practitioners and their employing healthcare institutions in various occupational and professional capacities, (d) amongst healthcare institutions in various operations that could characterize their modes of service delivery, and (e) between healthcare institutions and third-party affiliates providing outsourced/subsidiary services to support healthcare operations. Therefore, the regulation of healthcare information technologies also seeks to attribute the liabilities that must be accepted by the various healthcare stakeholders that feature in such interactions.

eHealth brings in several uncertainties to the business of healthcare service delivery, which regulation sometimes struggles to keep pace with. On the one hand, there is the duty of safeguarding ethical imperatives for healthcare subjects in a context where remote capabilities impose a capacity for anonymity, and expose service delivery channels and resources to a global scope of external interference that could be maliciously intended. Thus, creating a challenge for fairly attributing culpability for contravention in the absence of a globally acceptable/trans-jurisdictional legal framework, and sometimes also complicating the scope of healthcare regulation by dragging it across other domains like consumer protection, legal liability, and civil rights.

Then, on the other hand, there is the duty of monitoring the practices and operations of various stakeholders in the healthcare industry, to ensure that certain players (either through dominance that is created by ordinary market forces, or by way of consolidating interests and assets through mergers and acquisitions) do not exercise an outsized influence over the industry, which could ultimately endanger the interests of other stakeholders. Thereby, creating a situation wherein healthcare regulation has to grapple with certain intricacies of economics, market capitalization, competition law, and corporate governance.

Indeed, a number of such complexities have frequently been encountered in the course of regulating the operations, processes, and services of healthcare information and communication technologies (or, eHealth).

For example, consent is an extricability of personal healthcare and medical records, particularly due to the sensitive nature of data and information that applies in this context. But then, in the sense that eHealth is able to serve the best interests of the patients only to the extent that data and information about them are available for processing in order to inform the delivery of quality healthcare and medical services, regulation faces another challenge. This is the challenge of balancing the ethics of informed consent in a way that does not diminish the utilities afforded by eHealth for quality healthcare and medical services, which are also in the best interest of the data subjects (patients).

Again, there is the well-known challenge that frequently emerges when the rights to data privacy collide with the interests of public health and safety. In general, acceptable practices for the handling personal data require that the purposes for which data are collected, stored, and processed are very well-defined, transparent, and authorized by the patients (who are the data subjects in applications of eHealth) such that whenever data have to be processed or applied for a different purpose than that for which it was originally collected, then it is either that authorization is received again from the data subjects, or the data are collected again.

Yet, there are critical instances when the welfare and safety of the larger public might depend on processing sensitive personal data (such as for contact tracing during disease outbreaks, for security profiling, or for purposes that relate to legal proceedings), which had otherwise been collected for a different purpose that was well-defined and authorized at the time. Part of the goals of regulation is being able to balance such public interest against the imperatives of safeguarding sensitive healthcare and medical data that are collected, stored, and processed for enhancing service delivery in eHealth.

But then again, with growing tides of interference of sovereign political interests in the duties and responsibilities of healthcare delivery, both at the national and international levels, it sometimes poses a considerable challenge to clearly understand and delineate what might constitute public interest, especially when it involves the authoritarian/autocratic whims and caprices of an incumbent government being imposed on the polity. In this regard, regulation faces the challenge of clearly stipulating the circumstances under which it otherwise becomes permissible to subvert the need for authorization by data subjects, and apply eHealth data and medical records for other purposes that might be in the interest of the larger public, while also ensuring that such stipulations are safeguarded from being hijacked for political reasons that might be masquerading as public interest.

Also, there is the concern of being able to transmit eHealth data and information across borders for the purpose of enhancing the quality of medical services available to data subjects (patients), whereas these other jurisdictions could be subject to an entirely different body of laws for data protection, consumer protection, and legal liability. Thus, another goal of eHealth regulation is to establish a body of principles and specifications that work in harmony with existing laws across several jurisdictions, with minimum conflict.

The healthcare industry is one that is in an almost constant state of metamorphosis. Reflected by regular advancements in healthcare and medical procedures, which result in novel practices and applications that require regulatory oversight, the always-expanding scope of operations and service delivery that necessitate periodic reviews of existing regulation, frequent emergence of innovations (such as the Internet of things) that reveal new use cases and purposes wherein specification and standardization are needed, as well as mergers and acquisitions that require regulatory scrutiny and possible restructuring of ownership structures.

Together, all of these realities directly and indirectly impact the goals of regulation with respect to eHealth, sometimes creating new challenges or complicating existing ones. Regardless, the regulation of eHealth remains indispensable to preserving the utilities that eHealth offers for modern healthcare delivery in such a dynamic and complicated landscape.

Notable International Legislations

Certain International Legislations have been useful in helping to elucidate the context of some of the challenges that regulations face in trying to meet the goals of clarifying the nature, establishing the extent, and safeguarding the integrity of interactions that involve eHealth systems and applications for global healthcare service delivery. These international legislations attempt to define and specify best-practice standards, ethics, responsibilities, procedures, and operations across various aspects of healthcare service delivery wherever information and communication technologies are involved. These legislations are often situated and explored within a global framework of wider-acceptable considerations for safe, secure, ethical, and humanistic applications of eHealth.

Specifically, the WHO's Report on legal frameworks for eHealth[2] highlights two important International Legislations that are worth discussing. These are the Universal Declaration of Human Rights (UDHR)[3] of the United Nations, and the European Convention on Human Rights (ECHR)[4].

The UDHR, with specific reference to Article 12, specifies privacy as a universal human right. Declaring that "No one shall be subjected to arbitrary interference with his privacy, family, home or correspondence, nor to attacks upon his honour and reputation. Everyone has the right to the protection of the law against such interference or attacks". In this way, the responsibility and boundaries of jurisdictional regulations are established. This obligates such jurisdictional regulations to provide safeguards against the arbitrary invasion of personal privacy, while also taking care to ensure that the regulation itself does not contravene this very specification. This specification also emerges in Article 17 of another International Legislation known as the International Covenant on Civil and Political Rights (ICCPR)[5].

Indeed, Article 17 of the ICCPR gives more context to the provision of Article 12 of the UDHR through a General Comment (No. 16), which asserts that

> The gathering and holding of personal information on computers, data banks and other devices, whether by public authorities or private individuals or bodies, must be regulated by law. Effective measures have to be taken by States to ensure that information concerning a person's private life does not reach the hands of persons who are not authorized by law to receive,

process and use it, and is never used for purposes incompatible with the Covenant. In order to have the most effective protection of his private life, every individual should have the right to ascertain in an intelligible form, whether, and if so, what personal data is stored in automatic data files, and for what purposes. Every individual should also be able to, ascertain which public authorities or private individuals or bodies control or may control their files. If such files contain incorrect personal data or have been collected or processed contrary to the provisions of the law, every individual should have the right to request rectification or elimination.

Furthermore, Article 8 of the ECHR[6] also expands and builds upon this context by attributing a special status to personal medical and healthcare information. It recognizes that informed consent on the part of the data subject is critical to building and sustaining trust in the utility of eHealth for healthcare service delivery. It goes on to provide privacy safeguards with well-defined exceptions that could form legitimate grounds for bypassing consent of the data subject in access and processing personal medical/healthcare information.

These exceptions include when (1) data processing is in the vital interest of a patient, or of another individual who is physically or legally incapable of giving consent at the time, (2) the data processing is required for the purposes of preventive medicine, medical diagnosis, the provision of care or treatment, or the management of healthcare services and the personal data in question are processed by a health professional, and (3) there is substantial public interest or concern for public safety in the processing of personal medical/healthcare information, whereas, at least one of these criteria for exceptions must be met.

These notable international legislations have greatly helped to refine and filter the scope and context of regulatory responsibilities pertaining to contemporary issues of informed consent, privacy, identity and autonomy, and other digital rights that pertain to personal data. Indeed, they have inspired regulatory and legislative efforts that have emerged across various other regions, such as the African Union Convention on Cyber Security and Personal Data Protection: The Malabo Convention[7], and the African Declaration on Internet Rights and Freedoms[8], among others.

Roles & Responsibilities of Management and Administration

As previously highlighted, the roles and responsibilities of management and administration in healthcare organizations when it comes to eHealth, are often geared towards unifying the multi-stakeholder interests of governance, the imperatives of ethics, and the requirements of regulation, in a way that aligns eHealth applications with business goals, while preserving its utility for healthcare service delivery. Now, how this is to be achieved has often proven to be the difficult part.

At the point of commencement in this regard, it is important that healthcare organizations take an opportunity to evaluate the potentials and prospects that eHealth presents for business continuity, and then decide on what healthcare information and communication technologies, tools, and resources present the most important benefits to the success of their business model. For instance, in managing records for a large client base, it becomes infeasible and ineffective in the long run to perpetuate a manual (paper-based) records management model. In the same vein, as outpatient services begin to expand, it might become necessary to consider provisioning healthcare services in a way that is accessible to patients, even outside the healthcare facility.

These are possible considerations for enhancing effectiveness in business continuity, which might inform the decision of healthcare organizations to adopt healthcare information and communication technologies. But then, it is also critical at this point to ensure that the nitty-gritty pertaining to data, infrastructure, systems & devices, people & users, regulatory compliance, as well as other operational best practices for ethics, security, risk & incident management, and technical support that apply in such regards, are circumspectly considered.

Because data are frequently collected for various purposes at virtually every stage in the healthcare process when eHealth is applied, it is the responsibility of the management and administration of healthcare organizations to establish frameworks for keeping these data safe and ensuring that their invariants (Integrity, Confidentiality, and Availability) are preserved at all times. To this end, healthcare organizations should evaluate the data and information needs that are applicable to the various eHealth products and services that they provide, and then establish measures to safely acquire, organize/

process, store, transmit, and apply such data and information. When aspects of these operations are outsourced to vendors, affiliates, and subsidiaries, the parent healthcare organizations are equally responsible for ensuring that these partnering/affiliate organizations are held accountable to the same standards and best practices that they are themselves accountable to.

The manner in which this is done also has implications for the effectiveness of the service delivery processes and operations of healthcare organizations, as well as how efficiently the organizations' business model is able to meet the goals of investment. It could help healthcare organizations to forestall problems of liability that could have an impact on finances; prevent disruptions to operational regimens that could carry both reputational and legal consequences; respond effectively to regulation, innovation, and other advancements in a dynamic eHealth landscape; effectively allocate scarce resources to parallel business interests; and safeguard the ethical imperatives that are necessary for building consumer trust in eHealth products and services.

In addition, management and administration have frequently been held liable for technical and non-technical (including human) errors that occur in the processes and operations of eHealth products and service delivery. Thus, healthcare organizations have a role and responsibility in streamlining, scaling, and organizing the processes and operations of the eHealth products and services that they deploy in their chain – taking into cognizance the applicable environmental, socio-technical, and socio-cultural influences – to measure up to the accompanying risk and security implications. Sometimes, this may involve gauging their risk appetite, and measuring it against their technical and legal capacity, in order to better understand how capable they are in preventing eventualities, and how prepared they are to respond effectively when such eventualities occur before establishing adequate measures and mechanisms to mitigate the business impact of these eventualities.

Furthermore, management and administration have the added duty of ensuring a seamless coordination between the healthcare and medical professionals that use eHealth products and services, as well as the eHealth products and services that they use, especially when decision support purposes are within the scope of intentions.

This is important because critical implications for clinical decision support that is based on accurate and reliable data and information could be exacerbated by disparities in point-of-care medical and healthcare information, arising from errors that could be traced to man-made sources or machine defects. This situation is able to threaten the business interests of the healthcare organization with damning consequences.

Ultimately, it is the role and responsibility of healthcare managers and administrators to provide the leadership, structures, and frameworks, as well as establish the principles and processes that are needed to ensure that the utilities that eHealth offers for healthcare service delivery within their organizations are preserved in a way that is compliant with the requirements of the regulation, aligned with those well-known ethical considerations that inspire greater adoption of eHealth, and blends the various interests of multi-stakeholder governance.

For healthcare organizations to succeed in this regard, it is important to prioritize Information Technology assets in the business continuity plan. This way, eHealth products and services become key considerations for business continuity, so that they receive the measure of attention of Management and Administration that is needed to preserve their utility for quality healthcare service delivery. Research-driven enhancements and improvements would then become possible, so that eHealth products and services can continue to develop and advance internally, in ways that could positively influence returns on investment.

Compliance versus Security

It is important to recognize the danger of mistaking compliance with best practices and minimum requirements of third-party industry-wide contracts, for the existence of effective security across corporate or organizational levels. Whereas several regulations and widely recognized industry contracts have helped to specify minimum requirements, best practices, and voluntary standards that can be robustly considered for effective eHealth deployments, these must never be considered a substitute or alternative to the imperative of establishing clear organizational security policies and goals and putting in place the necessary technical processes, controls, systems, tools, and procedures for safeguarding the critical information and communication technology assets of the healthcare organization.

Unfortunately, it is becoming increasingly commonplace in the global healthcare industry to find medical institutions and healthcare organizations that have the compliance endorsements of various reputable third-party standards organizations, still succumb to cyber incidents and attacks in very embarrassing ways. This has often been traced to the absence of robust and effective security frameworks, even though compliance with multiple voluntary standards and best practices was very obvious.

Whereas *Compliance* simply represents the extent to which an organization has adhered to her contractual or operational obligations to third-party organizations (which could be industry standards bodies, regulatory authorities, etc.), *Security* entails moving beyond compliance to integrate the necessary technical processes, controls, systems, tools, and procedures that are needed to robustly and effectively safeguard critical digital electronic assets in alignment with clearly defined organizational goals.

However, in some contexts, compliance and security could often overlap. But even then, they do differ in their motives, scope, and goals. For all intents and purposes, the compliance requirements and obligations that healthcare organizations have to comply with are often blind to what constitutes the organization's goals and operational model, because they are typically geared towards building or sustaining public trust in the utilities that an industry has to offer. Thus, these compliance requirements and obligations have sometimes been discovered to be ambiguous and lacking in specifics. Rightly so, because they are often developed with a focus on an industry/industries in general, and not on any organization in particular.

Therefore, the onus is on medical institutions and healthcare organizations to move beyond meeting the duties of compliance to ensuring the imperatives of security across the entire information and communication technology assets and infrastructure of the organization.

Final Thoughts

As digital information and communications technologies continue to pervade the domain of global healthcare, finding practical application in the modern deployments of eHealth for healthcare service delivery, it is important that medical institutions and healthcare organizations are aware of, and prepared for the security implications and corporate liabilities that come with the adoption and usage of such technologies.

For the non-technical healthcare stakeholders (medical professionals, healthcare workers, regulatory and compliance agencies, health centre managers, administrators & insurers, clients/patients, and third-party vendors) who typically lack in-depth technical competence in the practical workings and operations of eHealth systems and infrastructures, and without sophisticated knowledge of the procedures and best practices for effective cybersecurity, the information in this Book would be useful in equipping them with the practical knowledge and insights that are needed to navigate the everyday realities and challenges of cybersecurity in the delivery of healthcare services.

However, it is necessary to stress that at organizational/corporate levels, it is important that adopting and applying the information and recommendations provided in this book are done in consultation with technical experts and professionals who would help guide and contextualize these information and recommendations to align with the operational realities and goals of the organization. The importance of this cannot be exaggerated.

Furthermore, it is hoped that the book would also have some appeal for (cybersecurity) enthusiasts generally and even in the affiliated/adjoining sectors of global healthcare, who are looking to have a foundational understanding of the cybersecurity threats and risks that pertain to the healthcare sector, while also providing a useful utility for facilitators and instructors who design, create, and facilitate training programs in healthcare information technologies, either as part of formal medical/nursing school degree, certificate, or diploma training, or as post-qualification continuing education programs in healthcare, medicine, public health, or nursing.

In addition, it is also expected that the language, structure, and design of the Book would resonate with Medical Boards, Nursing Councils, Public Health Professional Societies, and other Healthcare Bodies/Associations at national and regional (or international) levels. In this regard, it is anticipated that success would come on the heels of the reality that while the subject area remains one that is of much contemporary relevance, the short supply of rudimentary training resources targeting non-technical audiences poses an obstacle to the effectiveness of training programs in the subject domain. It is within this gap that this Book has provided a befitting resource that is relevant to the reality and necessities of this problem.

But ultimately, armed with the broad insights and perspectives provided in this Book, which have been accumulated from across several organizational and national contexts, it is hoped that healthcare stakeholders who seek to do their part towards quelling the tides of cyber incidents and attacks that continue to destabilize the global healthcare industry would find a useful and practical guide for progress and success in this pursuit.

Notes

1 World Health Organization (WHO) (n.d.). *eHealth Governance*. https://www.who.int/ehealth/governance/en/
2 Wilson, P. (2012). Legal frameworks for eHealth. *Global Observatory for eHealth series – Volume 5*. World Health Organization (WHO). https://www.who.int/goe/publications/legal_framework_web.pdf
3 United Nations (2015). *Universal Declaration of Human Rights (UDHR)*. https://www.un.org/en/udhrbook/pdf/udhr_booklet_en_web.pdf
4 Council of Europe (2013, October 02). *European Convention on Human Rights*. https://www.echr.coe.int/documents/convention_eng.pdf
5 United Nations (1966). *International Covenant on Civil and Political Rights*. UN Office of the High Commissioner on Human Rights. https://www.ohchr.org/en/professionalinterest/pages/ccpr.aspx
6 Council of Europe (2020, December 31). *Guide on Article 8 of the European Convention on Human Rights*. European Court of Human Rights. https://www.echr.coe.int/documents/guide_art_8_eng.pdf
7 The African Union Commission (2014, June 27). *African Union Convention on Cyber Security and Personal Data Protection*. https://au.int/en/treaties/african-union-convention-cyber-security-and-personal-data-protection
8 Orrell, T. (2015, November). *The African Declaration on Internet Rights and Freedoms: A Positive Agenda for Human Rights Online*. Global Partners Digital. https://www.gp-digital.org/wp-content/uploads/pubs/african-declaration-a-positive-agenda-for-rights-online.pdf

Glossary of Definitions

Access Authentication: An access control measure that requires authorized entities to confirm or verify their person and identity by providing certain information (that is usually confidential or unique), prior to gaining access to a system or network.

Access Control: These are measures that are put in place to restrict entry and engagement with a system or network to only such entities that are authorized.

Anonymization: The practice of removing all personally identifiable information from a body of data, such that it becomes impossible to identify the original data subject(s) by any means at all.

Anti-malware: A device or application that provides protection against various malware.

Bot: A software program, device, or system that is able to receive, process, and execute commands/instructions, such that enable it to perform pre-defined tasks and operations in a repetitive manner that can be automated.

Botnet: A collection of infected or compromised systems and devices that are under the control of an attacker, and can be deployed to perpetrate and amplify the impact of malicious operations against targets of interest.

Bring Your Own Device (BYOD): A working arrangement that permits employees of an organization to bring and use personal devices and systems within the corporate environment, and also gain access to organizational digital resources and platforms using these personal devices and systems.

Code: A collection of instructions written in a particular computational language, which describes/specifies the procedures and operations that would be undertaken in the execution/processing of a particular task. It is otherwise referred to as "*Source Code*".

Credentials: Digital artefacts that contain the information needed to prove or verify something about the subject or user that holds such credentials.

Cross-Site Scripting: Written as "XSS" in shorthand, it is a security vulnerability of web applications that allows malicious actors to compromise or interfere with the legitimate interactions that authorized users have with such applications.

Cryptanalytics: It generally refers to the science, procedures, technologies, and activities that are applied in an analysis aimed at understanding the hidden aspects of information systems and technologies, to enable the encryption and decryption of messages without the use of secret keys.

Cyber-Attack: A criminal offence against a digital information technology asset (networks, devices, systems, etc.) that seeks to gain unauthorized access, control, and usage of such asset for malicious purposes. It typically features a range of tools, techniques, methodologies, and strategies.

Cyber-Physical Systems: An implementation that involves the use of computers in monitoring physical phenomena, and/or controlling physical processes and operations, featuring the use of sensors (to detect events as impulses and variations in the physical environment), and actuators (to take actions in response to detections).

Cybersecurity: The practice and profession of defending information technology systems and assets against threats, malicious actors, and attacks.

Data Breach: A cyber incident that intentionally or unwittingly results in the compromise of security, leading to unauthorized access, disclosure, or theft of information that is considered valuable and confidential, and should be otherwise secured.

Data Element: The atomicity of data that is defined in semantics and representation, and has a value that can be collected, processed, stored, or transmitted.

Data Invariant: An unchanging property that is binding on a functional body of data, and all operations that are performed on such data – before, during, and/or after collection, processing, storage, or transmission.

Data Subject: A human or non-human entity, to which a particular data element refers.

Denial of Service: The malicious action of preventing legitimate users from accessing digital platforms, utilities, and resources (e.g., systems, devices, and networks), typically by flooding and engaging such digital platforms, utilities, and resources with useless (sometimes malicious) traffic and requests.

Digital Footprint: Information that is available about an individual by virtue of their online presence and activities on the Internet.

Digital Shadow: The collection of all residual information (confidential, proprietary, or sensitive) about an individual, which is left behind following engagements with a digital service or platform.

Domain Name: A string that perpetually identifies (that is, names and addresses) an online location as one that is autonomous in its administration, authority, and control.

Encryption: The process of encoding sensitive information in such a way that it can only be accessed and understood by authorized entities that possess the information that is needed to reverse the encoding operation (through a process known as decryption). A secret key is a critical component in the process of encryption and decryption, and holds the necessary information for successfully and legitimately encoding and decoding data.

End-to-End (E2E): A design principle which ensures that the features and functions that are critical to application or security operations reside in the nodes sitting at both ends of a medium that serves as an intermediary between these end nodes for the purpose of communication or exchange.

Enumeration: An attack step that seeks to gather relevant information with the aim of deducing a complete or representative listing/profile of the entities of interest within a target domain/environment, which is often a computer network, a physical office location, or a computer system.

Firewall: A computer program that provides defence against unauthorized access to computer systems or private networks.

Information and Communication Technologies (ICTs): A broad terminology that is typically applied to describe the unified models, frameworks, and apparatuses for communication and information exchange, as well as the integral role played by computers and other digital electronic devices in facilitating storage, manipulation, transmission, retrieval, and access to such information.

Input Validation: A control mechanism that is built into a device or software to check and ensure that data entered by users meet the format, specifications, and requirements for processing.

Keylogger: Hardware or software that is able to monitor and record user keystrokes that are delivered through input devices to a digital computing system or platform, and then store or relay such information to an attacker. It is usually used to steal sensitive information for malicious purposes.

Login Timeout: A security configuration that allows users to be automatically logged out from digital systems, devices, and applications after a certain time period has elapsed.

Malware: A portmanteau collocation of the terms "MALicious" and "softWARE". Referring to computer programs that are designed to infiltrate digital systems and networks without consent or authorization, and often with the capacity to cause damage.

Man-in-the-Middle: The practice of intercepting digital communications by interposing between two unknowing entities, often with malicious intent to relay, re-route, alter, or simply gain (otherwise) unauthorized access to information/data.

Minimization: The practice of limiting data collection operations to receiving only such data elements that are necessary and relevant to fulfilling a specific purpose that is well-defined.

Network: An interconnection of digital electronic devices (such as computers) that enables communication/information exchange, and the sharing of files and resources over electronic channels.

Network Protocol: The rules of engagement that define and specify how data and information exchange would take place between devices within a computer network.

Network Sniffer: A software or device that enables the real-time monitoring and analysis of packets and protocols on a network for legitimate or malicious purposes. It is sometimes also referred to as a network analyser.

Packet: The unit of data that is carried by a network, and is formatted to contain the necessary information and control parameters that are needed to transmit the data across the network.

Packet Tracer: A software or device that is used to map the path along which packets travel on a network, often by imitating or simulating the layout and structure of the network at the physical, logical, or conceptual level.

Patch: An enhancement that is provided for a computer program, or the files and data that it uses, in order to fix security vulnerabilities or insufficiencies in the program.

Phishing: A form of Social Engineering that usually involves an attacker/malicious individual posing as a trusted entity in a text-based communication (e.g., email, instant message [IM], short message [SMS], etc.).

Platform: A business utility with an operating model that allows multiple participants (consumers) to connect to it for the purposes of interacting, sharing, creating, and deriving value typically through dyadic engagements and exchanges.

Policy: A targeted body of procedures and principles that are established to provide guidelines for informed decision-making and actions that lead to rational outcomes, which are in line with broader envisioned goals.

Programming: The process/task of creating solutions to computational problems through instructions or commands written in a particular language that can be understood and processed by a computer system.

Pseudonymization: The practice of substituting personally identifiable information in a body of data with non-identifiable information mapped to a description that enables the original personal information to be easily deduced; thus, transforming the original data into one that does not personally identify data subjects any longer.

Reconnaissance: A preliminary step in an attack procedure that seeks to gather useful information about the identities, operations, and vulnerabilities in target systems/networks (sometimes referred to as enumeration), often with the aim of exploiting such vulnerabilities in a later attack against the system/network.

Scavenging: The practice of scouring through garbage for residual information of interest; which, although, might have been ordinarily inaccessible (due to its sensitive nature), could provide useful intelligence for future malicious operations.

Secure Socket Communication: A protocol that is used to encrypt web communications/transactions. It is sometimes also referred to as *Secure Socket Layer (SSL) Communication.*

Security Protocol: The sets and sequences of processes and operations that are put in place for the purpose of preserving security and ensuring other security-related functions.

Server: A hardware or software computing system that functions primarily to provide utility and services to other programs, systems, and devices (often referred to as "clients") that connect to it.

Shoulder Surfing: The practice of spying on users by looking over their shoulders as they use applications or digital electronic devices, often with the motive of learning sensitive user information (such as usernames, passwords, secure URLs, etc.).

Smash 'n' Grab: An operation that involves a malicious actor quickly smashing through a security or other barriers to lay a hold on valuables.

Social Engineering: The usually malicious practice of posing as a trusted entity in order to deceive individuals/users into taking actions or divulging (sensitive) information that they might otherwise not have been inclined to.

Spoofing: The often-malicious impersonation of an authorized entity in digital communications, in order to attain/receive/transfer the privileges, benefits, and utilities provided to the authorized entity by a system or network. It is a form of digital identity theft.

Subversion: The malicious process of bypassing or over-running the control and security functions of a digital computing system or resource, often for the purpose of gaining unauthorized access and control.

Tailgating: The practice of gaining unauthorized access to a usually secure or restricted location/facility as a result of bypassing physical security and access control measures or systems by tagging closely enough to someone with authorized access. It is otherwise referred to as *Piggybacking*.

Threat Actors: Human or non-human individual or group entities that seek to compromise the security of computer systems or networks for malicious purposes.

Threat Landscape: An anthology of threats that are native to a specific context or domain, about which it is known what risks they present, what assets they target, what actors are involved, and the trends they manifest.

Transloading: The process of transferring or translocating a usually malicious digital payload between or across systems, devices, networks, or other digital information technology media.

Two-Factor Authentication: A form of authentication that requires authorized users to present more than one type of information for identity confirmation/verification, prior to gaining access to a system or network.

Uniform Resource Locator (URL): An identifier that references a resource on a local network, or on the World Wide Web/Internet. It is otherwise referred to as a web address.

Unstructured Supplementary Service Data (USSD): A protocol that enables users' mobile telephone devices to communicate with the computers of network operators/service providers using short codes that are otherwise referred to as "feature codes", or "quick codes", and usually involve special characters like "*" and "#".

Virtual Private Networks (VPNs): An encrypted connection that links a device to a network across the open Internet – providing a reliable means for transmitting data securely, without the risk of interference or interception.

Virus: A malware that propagates by binding itself to user and system files, and is able to inflict damage on digital systems or networks, according to the instructions contained in its program code.

Vishing: A form of Social Engineering that usually involves an attacker/malicious individual posing as a trusted entity in a voice-based communication (e.g., phone calls, audio messages, etc.).

Wardriving: The act of locating wireless network access points typically by driving around various locations, often with the aim of exploiting successful connections to such wireless access points for malicious purposes. It is sometimes referred to as Access Point Mapping.

Website: A collection of web pages that feature related content about a person, organization, concept, technology, or other entity/phenomenon; and is tied to a particular name (known as a domain name) that makes it discoverable on the Internet.

Bibliography

European Commission (2014, July 23). *Overview of the national laws on electronic health records in the EU Member States and their interaction with the provision of cross-border eHealth services.* https://ec.europa.eu/health/sites/health/files/ehealth/docs/laws_report_recommendations_en.pdf

European Union Agency for Network and Information Security (ENISA) (2015). *Security and Resilience in eHealth: Security Challenges and Risks.* https://www.enisa.europa.eu/publications/security-and-resilience-in-ehealth-infrastructures-and-services/at_download/fullReport

Herveg, J., Silber, D., Van Doosselaere, C., & Wilson, P. (2006). *Deliverable 5: Final Recommendations on Legal Issues in eHealth. Study on Legal and Regulatory Aspects of eHealth: "Legally eHealth".* http://ehma.org/wordpress/wp-content/uploads/2016/08/Legally_eHealth-Del_05-Recommendations2.pdf

International Development Research Centre (IDRC) (2010, December). *Electronic Health Privacy and Security in Developing Countries and Humanitarian Operations.* Policy Engagement Network for the IDRC. The London School of Economics and Political Science. http://personal.lse.ac.uk/martinak/eHealth.pdf

Miesperä, A., Ahonen, S. M., & Reponen, J. (2013). Ethical aspects of eHealth-systematic review of open access articles. *Finnish Journal of eHealth and eWelfare*, 5(4), 165–171. https://journal.fi/finjehew/article/view/9401/6707

Salvi, M. (2012, February 22). *Ethics of Information and Communication Technologies.* Publications Office of the EU. https://op.europa.eu/en/publication-detail/-/publication/c35a8ab5-a21d-41ff-b654-8cd6d41f6794

Sembok, T. M. (November 2003). *Ethics of Information Communication Technology (ICT). Proceedings of the Regional Meeting on Ethics of Science and Technology* (pp. 239-325). Bangkok: UNESCO – Regional Unit for Social & Human Sciences in Asia and the Pacific (RUSHSAP).

Townsend, B. A. (2017, March). Privacy and Data Protection in eHealth in Africa: An assessment of the regulatory frameworks that govern privacy and data protection in the effective implementation of electronic health care in Africa: Is there a need for reform and greater regional collaboration in regulatory policymaking? Doctoral Thesis. Cape Town, South Africa: University of Cape Town. https://open.uct.ac.za/bitstream/handle/11427/25510/thesis_law_2017_townsend_beverley_alice.pdf

Wilson, P. (2012). Legal frameworks for eHealth. *Global Observatory for eHealth series - Volume 5.* World Health Organization (WHO). https://www.who.int/goe/publications/legal_framework_web.pdf

World Health Organization (WHO) (2016). *Monitoring and Evaluating Digital Health Interventions: A practical guide to conducting research and assessment.* https://apps.who.int/iris/bitstream/handle/10665/252183/9789241511766-eng.pdf

Printed in the United States
by Baker & Taylor Publisher Services